Student Workbook for

Phlebotomy Essentials

Fifth Edition

Ruth E. McCall, BS, MT (ASCP)
Retired Program Director and Instructor
Central New Mexico Community College
Albuquerque, New Mexico

Cathee M. Tankersley, BS, MT (ASCP)
President, NuHealth Educators, LLC
Faculty, Emeritus
Phoenix College
Phoenix, Arizona

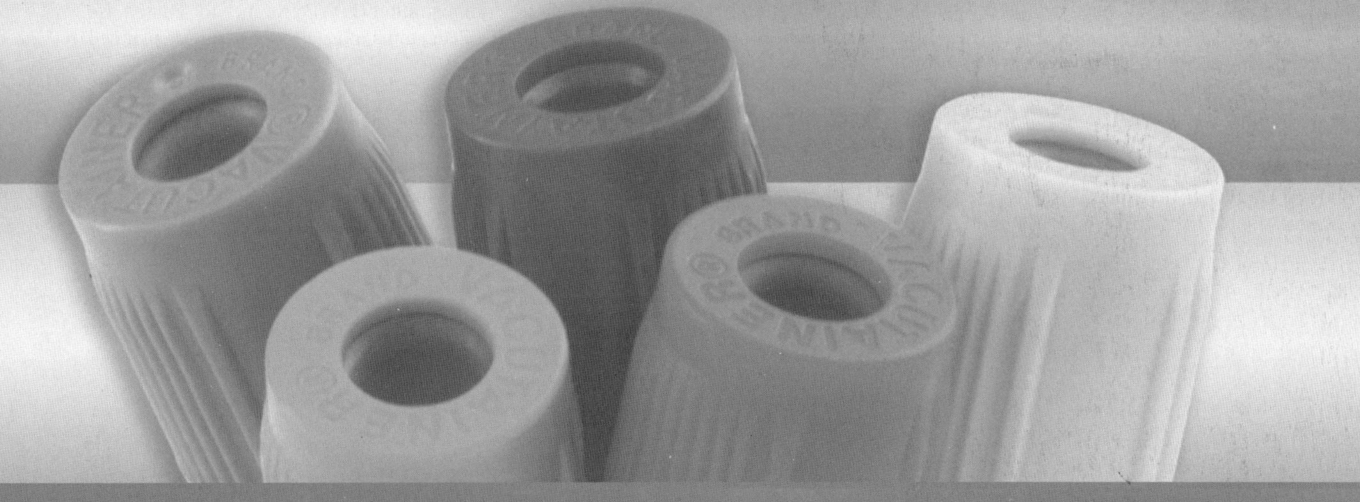

Wolters Kluwer Health | Lippincott Williams & Wilkins
Philadelphia • Baltimore • New York • London
Buenos Aires • Hong Kong • Sydney • Tokyo

Acquisitions Editor: Peter Sabatini
Product Manager: Meredith L. Brittain
Marketing Manager: Shauna Kelley
Designer: Holly McLaughlin
Production Services: Aptara, Inc.

Fifth Edition

351 West Camden Street
Baltimore, MD 21201

Two Commerce Square
2001 Market Street
Philadelphia, PA 19103

Printed in China

9 8 7 6

DISCLAIMER

Care has been taken to confirm the accuracy of the information present and to describe generally accepted practices. However, the authors, editors, and publisher are not responsible for errors or omissions or for any consequences from application of the information in this book and make no warranty, expressed or implied, with respect to the currency, completeness, or accuracy of the contents of the publication. Application of this information in a particular situation remains the professional responsibility of the practitioner; the clinical treatments described and recommended may not be considered absolute and universal recommendations.

The authors, editors, and publisher have exerted every effort to ensure that drug selection and dosage set forth in this text are in accordance with the current recommendations and practice at the time of publication. However, in view of ongoing research, changes in government regulations, and the constant flow of information relating to drug therapy and drug reactions, the reader is urged to check the package insert for each drug for any change in indications and dosage and for added warnings and precautions. This is particularly important when the recommended agent is a new or infrequently employed drug.

Some drugs and medical devices presented in this publication have U.S. Food and Drug Administration (FDA) clearance for limited use in restricted research settings. It is the responsibility of the healthcare provider to ascertain the FDA status of each drug or device planned for use in their clinical practice.

To purchase additional copies of this book, call our customer service department at **(800) 638-3030** or fax orders to **(301) 223-2320**. International customers should call **(301) 223-2300**.

Visit Lippincott Williams & Wilkins on the Internet: http://www.lww.com. Lippincott Williams & Wilkins customer service representatives are available from 8:30 am to 6:00 pm, EST.

To all the students whom we have had the privilege of teaching and who have made our teaching careers worthwhile.

RUTH E. McCALL

CATHEE M. TANKERSLEY

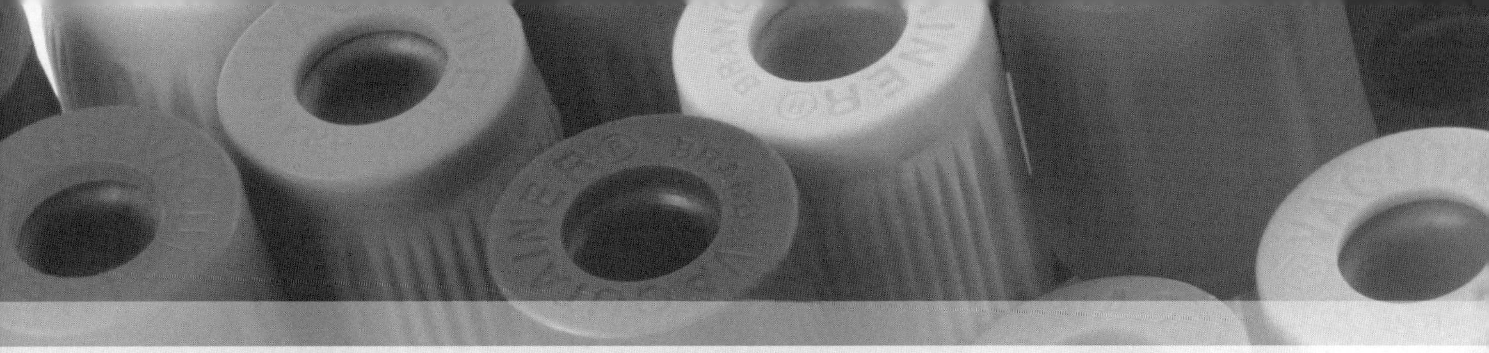

Preface

Student Workbook for Phlebotomy Essentials, fifth edition, is designed to be used in combination with the fifth edition of the *Phlebotomy Essentials* textbook as a valuable learning resource that will help the student master the principles of phlebotomy by reinforcing key concepts and procedures covered in the textbook. The workbook offers a variety of exercises and tools to make it easy and fun for the student to understand and remember essential information and enhance critical-thinking skills.

Some exercises require written answers to provide spelling practice in addition to testing knowledge. Every chapter includes:

- **Chapter Objectives** that correspond to those in the companion textbook
- **Matching Activities** including Key Term Matching
- **Labeling Activities** to help students visualize important material
- **Knowledge Drills** including fun scrambled word activities
- **Skills Drills**, including requisition and procedure practice activities
- **Chapter and Unit Crossword Puzzles** to help make learning fun
- **Chapter Review Questions** to test comprehension of chapter material
- **Case Studies** to bring concepts to life

Answers to all workbook activities and exercises are located in the Faculty Resource Center at http://thepoint.lww.com/McCallWorkbook5e. Access to these answers is strictly limited to faculty only. If you have further questions concerning this workbook, please email customerservice@lww.com.

The authors sincerely wish to express their gratitude to all who assisted in and supported this effort.

RUTH E. McCALL

CATHEE M. TANKERSLEY

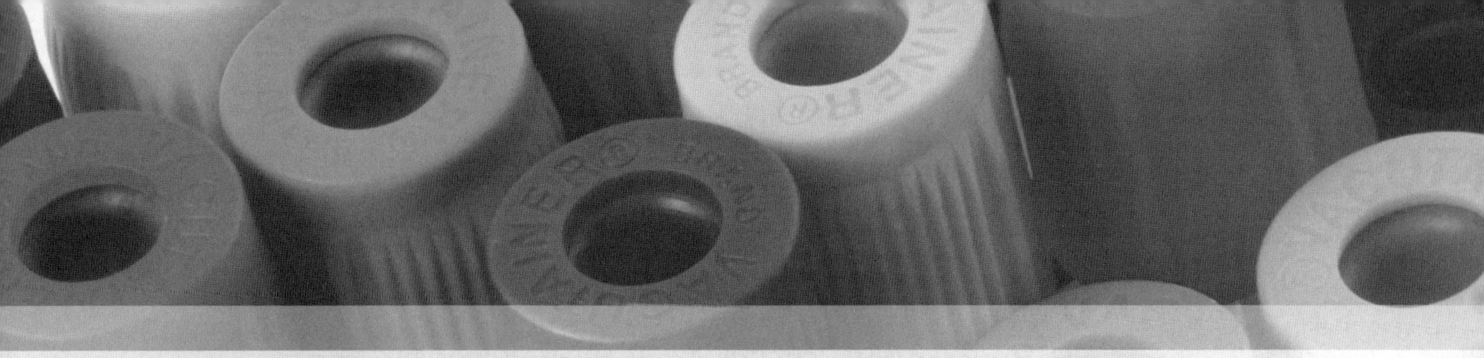

Reviewers

Diana Alagna, RN, RMA
Program Director
Medical Assisting
Branford Hall Career Institute
Southington, Connecticut

Gerry Brasin, AS, CMA (AAMA), CPC
Coordinator
Education/Compliance
Premier Education Group
Springfield, Massachuesetts

Konnie Briggs, LN
Instructor
Health Science
Houston Community College
Houston, Texas

Lou Brown, BS, MT (ASCP), CMA (AAMA)
Program Director
Medical Assisting and Phlebotomy
Wayne Community College
Goldsboro, North Carolina

Susen Edwards, MA
Program Coordinator
Allied Health
Middlesex County College
Edison, New Jersey

Lance Everett, BA, CPT
Director
Allied Health
National Career Education
Rancho Cordova, California

Nancy Feulner, MS Ed
Program Coordinator
Health Science
College of DuPage
Glen Ellyn, Illinois

Kathleen Finnegan, MS, MT (ASCP), SH
Clinical Associate Professor and Chair
Clinical Laboratory Sciences
Stony Brook University
Stony Brook, New York

Tammy Gallagher, BS, MT
Medical Technologist
Butler County Community College
Butler, Pennsylvania

Henry Gomez, MD
Associate Professor
Division of Health Disciplines
ASA Institute
Brooklyn, New York

Cheryl Milish, AAS
Instructor
Allied Health
Southwestern College
Florence, Kentucky

Judith Miller, BS, MT (ASCP)
Clinical Coordinator
Medical Laboratory Technician Program
Barton County Community College
Great Bend, Kansas

Lane Miller, MBA/HCM
Director
Continuing Education
Medical Careers Institute
Virginia Beach, Virginia

Carole Mullins, BS, MT (ASCP), MPA, DLM (ASCP)
Adjunct Faculty
Nursing and Human Services
Southwestern Michigan College
Dowagiac, Michigan

Michael Murphy, CMA (AAMA)
Program Coordinator
Berdan Institute at The Summit Medical Group
Union, New Jersey

Debbie Reasoner, (NHA)-CPT-CHI
Director and Instructor
Phlebotomy/Lab Assistant
West Coast Phlebotomy, Inc.
Oregon City, Oregon

Marie Thomas, CLT, CMA
Clinical Instructor/Lead
Medical Assisting
Berdan Institute
Wayne, New Jersey

Barbara Vaiden, BS, MT (ASCP)
Supervisor
Phlebotomy
OSF Saint Anthony Medical Center
Rockford, Illinois

Nicole Walton, PBT, RMA
Phlebotomy Instructor
Center for Workforce Development
College of Western Idaho
Boise, Idaho

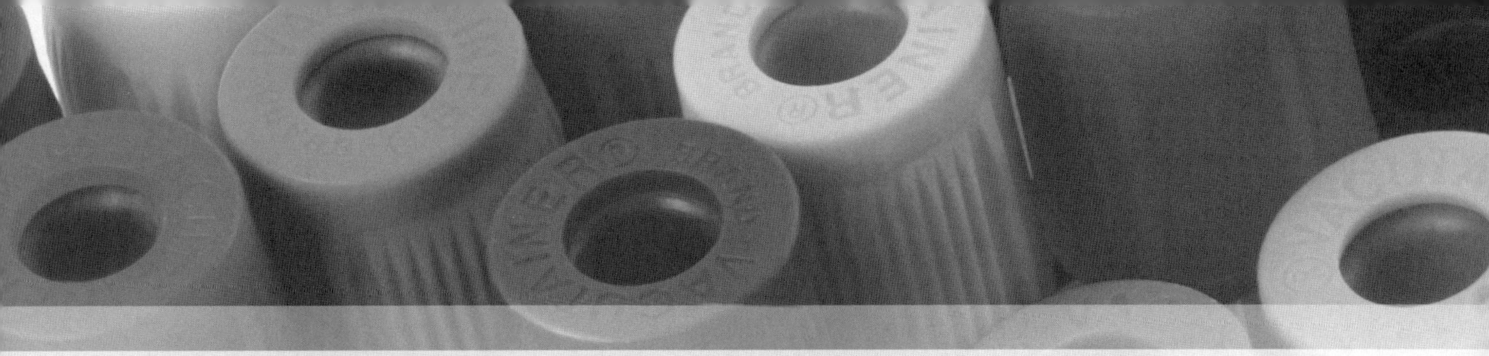

Contents

UNIT IV SPECIAL PROCEDURES 197

UNIT I INTRODUCTION TO PHLEBOTOMY IN HEALTHCARE

CHAPTER 1

Phlebotomy: Past and Present and the Healthcare Setting

OBJECTIVES

Study the information in your textbook that corresponds to each objective to prepare yourself for the activities in this chapter.

1. Define the key terms and abbreviations listed at the beginning of this chapter.
2. Describe the evolution of phlebotomy and the role of the phlebotomist in today's healthcare setting.
3. Describe the traits that form the professional image and identify national organizations that support professional recognition of phlebotomists.
4. Describe the basic concepts of communication as they relate to healthcare and how appearance and nonverbal messages affect the communication process.
5. Describe proper telephone protocol in a laboratory and other healthcare settings.
6. Demonstrate an awareness of the different types of healthcare settings.
7. Compare types of third-party payers, coverage, and methods of payment to the patient, provider, and institutions.
8. Describe traditional hospital organization and identify the healthcare providers in the inpatient facility.
9. List the clinical analysis areas of the laboratory and the types of laboratory procedures performed in the different areas
10. Describe the different levels of personnel found in the clinical laboratory and how the regulations of the Clinical Laboratory Improvement Amendment affect their job descriptions.

Matching

Use choices only once unless otherwise indicated.

MATCHING 1-1: KEY TERMS AND DESCRIPTIONS

Match the key term with the *best* description.

Key Terms (1–15)

1. ____ AHCCCS
2. ____ APC
3. ____ certification
4. ____ CLIA '88
5. ____ communication barriers
6. ____ CMS
7. ____ CPT
8. ____ case manager
9. ____ exsanguinate
10. ____ HIPAA
11. ____ HMOs
12. ____ ICD-9-CM
13. ____ IDS
14. ____ kinesic slip
15. ____ kinesics

Descriptions

A. Evidence that an individual has mastered fundamental competencies in a technical specialty
B. Health Insurance Portability and Accountability Act
C. Ambulatory patient classification
D. Experienced HC professional that serves as the patient's advocate and adviser
E. Verbal and nonverbal messages do not match
F. Health maintenance organizations
G. Arizona Health Care Cost Containment System
H. Current procedural terminology codes
I. Biases that are major obstructions to verbal communication.
J. *International Classification of Diseases,* 9th Revision, Clinical Modification
K. Clinical Laboratory Improvement Amendments of 1988
L. Remove all blood
M. Centers for Medicare and Medicaid Services
N. Integrated healthcare delivery system
O. Study of nonverbal communication

Match the key term with the *best* description.

Key Terms (16–30)

16. ____ MCOs
17. ____ Medicaid
18. ____ Medicare
19. ____ MLS
20. ____ PHI
21. ____ PHS
22. ____ phlebotomy
23. ____ polycythemia
24. ____ PPOs
25. ____ primary care
26. ____ proxemics
27. ____ reference laboratories
28. ____ secondary care
29. ____ tertiary care
30. ____ third-party payer

Descriptions

A. Care by physician who assumes ongoing responsibility for maintaining patients' health.
B. Care by specialist who can perform out-of-the-ordinary procedures in outpatient facilities
C. More recent term meaning venesection
D. Disorder involving overproduction of red blood cells
E. Highly complex care from practitioners in a hospital or overnight facility
F. Managed care organizations
G. Federally funded program that provides healthcare to seniors, 65 and older
H. Promotes and administers programs for public health
I. Federal and state program that provides medical assistance for eligible low-income Americans
J. Insurance company that pays for healthcare services on behalf of a patient
K. Preferred provider organizations
L. Study of an individual's concept and use of space
M. Large, independent laboratories that test specimens from many different facilities
N. Medical Laboratory Scientist
O. Protected health information

MATCHING 1-2: CERTIFICATION AGENCIES

Match the certification agency with the title awarded. *A title may be used more than once.*

Certification Agency

1. C American Society of Clinical Pathologists
2. A American Medical Technologists
3. D National Center for Competency Testing
4. B American Certification Agency
5. B National Healthcareer Association

Title Awarded

A. RPT
B. CPT
C. PBT
D. NCPT

MATCHING 1-3: METHODS OF PAYMENT AND DIAGNOSIS CODING

Match the methods of payment and diagnosis coding with the appropriate definition.

Method of Payment and Diagnosis Coding

1. _____ Ambulatory patient classification
2. _____ *International Classification of Diseases,* 9th Revision
3. _____ Prospective payment system
4. _____ Diagnosis-related groups

Definitions

A. Begun in 1983 to limit and standardize the Medicare/Medicaid payments made to hospitals
B. Reimburses healthcare facilities a set amount for each patient procedure using established disease categories
C. A classification system implemented in 2000 for determining payment to hospitals for outpatient service
D. All major payers use this coding system, which groups together similar disease and operations for reimbursement

MATCHING 1-4: LABORATORY TESTS AND DEPARTMENTS

Match the laboratory tests with the departments that perform them. *Departments can be used more than one time.*

Laboratory Tests

1. _____ BMP
2. _____ PT
3. _____ Hct
4. _____ WBC diff
5. _____ Nitrites
6. _____ ANA
7. _____ Specific gravity
8. _____ ALT
9. _____ D-dimer
10. _____ Triglycerides
11. _____ Blood culture
12. _____ EBV
13. _____ Type and Rh
14. _____ Gram stain
15. _____ DAT
16. _____ Troponin
17. _____ Bilirubin
18. _____ APTT
19. _____ Plt ct
20. _____ Glucose

Laboratory Departments

A. Hematology
B. Blood Bank
C. Coagulation
D. Chemistry
E. Immunology
F. Urinalysis
G. Microbiology
H. Histology
I. Cytology

MATCHING 1-5: PATIENT CONDITIONS AND MEDICAL SPECIALTIES

Match the specialties with types of patient conditions they serve.

Patient Conditions

1. ____ Tumors, benign and malignant
2. ____ Eye examinations
3. ____ Endocrine gland disorders
4. ____ Diseases of the heart
5. ____ Disorders of the brain and spinal cord
6. ____ Well checkups for children
7. ____ Kidney function
8. ____ Urinary tract disease
9. ____ Conditions of the skin
10. ____ Age-related disorders
11. ____ Digestive tract disorders
12. ____ Respiratory system conditions
13. ____ Inflammation and joint diseases
14. ____ Contagious, pathogenic infections
15. ____ Disorders of the blood

Medical Specialties

A. Anesthesiology
B. Cardiology
C. Dermatology
D. Endocrinology
E. Gastroenterology
F. Gerontology
G. Hematology
H. Infectious Diseases
I. Nephrology
J. Neurology
K. Oncology
M. Ophthalmology
N. Pediatrics
O. Psychiatry
P. Pulmonary Medicine
Q. Rheumatology

Labeling Exercises

LABELING 1-1: VERBAL COMMUNICATION BARRIERS

Using the TEXTBOOK, identify each HCW communication barrier in the numbered boxes on the left of the communication feedback loop diagram and each "Client" communication barrier on the right. Write the answers in the corresponding blanks below the diagram.

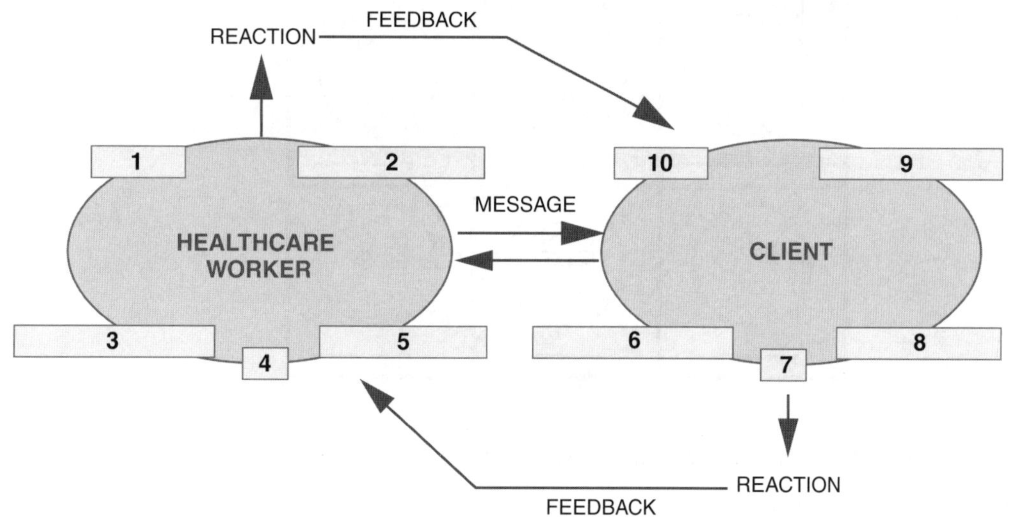

1. ______________________________

____

2. ______________________________

____

3. ______________________________

____

4. ______________________________

____

5. ______________________________

____

6. ______________________________

____

7. ______________________________

____

8. ______________________________

____

9. ______________________________

____

10. ______________________________

____

LABELING 1-2: NONVERBAL FACIAL CUES

Label each of the sketches below with the correct facial cue from the following list:

- Surprise
- Fear
- Sad
- Happy
- Anger
- Disgust

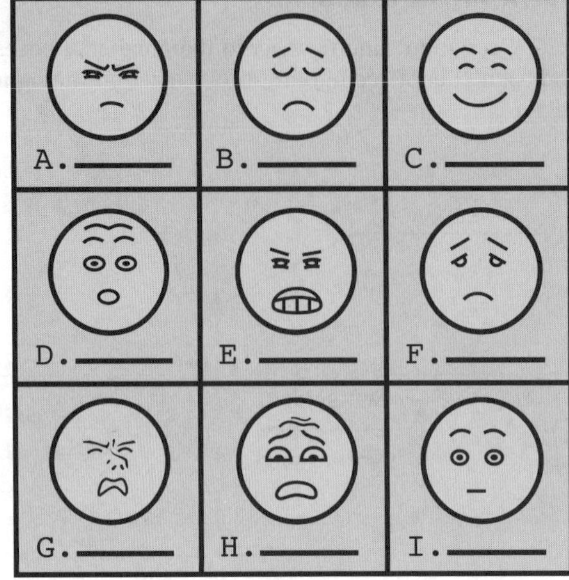

LABELING 1-3: HOSPITAL ORGANIZATIONAL CHART

Fill in the names of the major divisions in a typical hospital organizational chart.

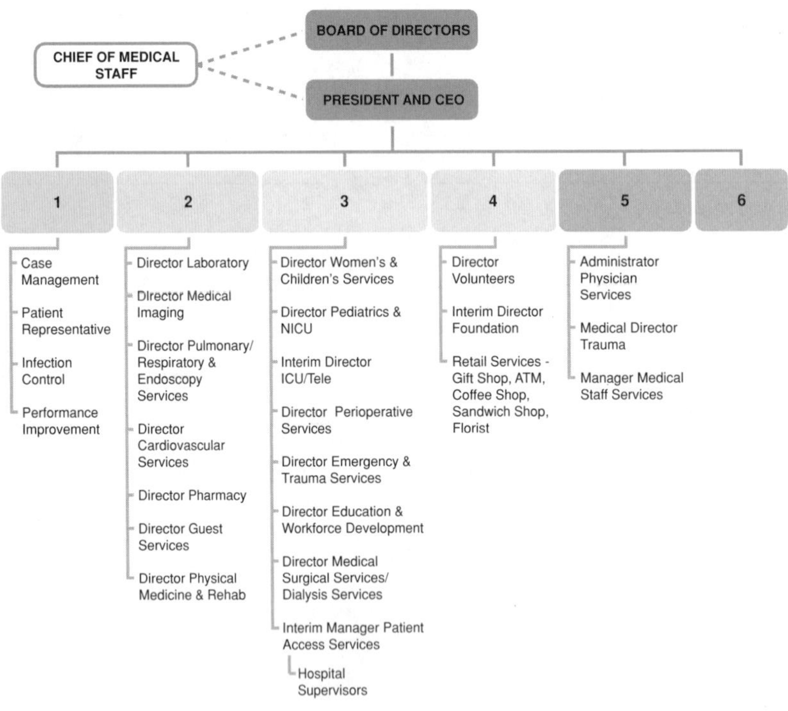

1. ______________________________
2. ______________________________
3. ______________________________
4. ______________________________
5. ______________________________
6. ______________________________

Knowledge Drills

KNOWLEDGE DRILL 1-1: CAUTION AND KEY POINT RECOGNITION

The following sentences have been taken from caution and key point statements found throughout Chapter 1 of the textbook. Using the TEXTBOOK, fill in the blanks with the missing information.

1. By recognizing (A) ______________, the phlebotomist promotes (B) ______________ and harmonious relationships that directly improve health (C) ______________, the (D) ______________ of services, and (E) ______________ relations.
2. Maintaining (A) ______________ is such an (B) ______________ issue in testing for (C) ______________ that the patient must sign a (D) ______________ before the specimen for the test can be collected.
3. To (A) ______________ effectively with someone, it is important to establish good (B) ______________. A patient or client may be made to (C) ______________ and more like an (D) ______________ rather than a human being if no eye contact is established.
4. Phlebotomists will find that when dealing with (A) ______________ who are (B) ______________ or (C) ______________, a confident and professional (D) ______________ will be most (E) ______________ to doing their job.

KNOWLEDGE DRILL 1-2: SCRAMBLED WORDS

Scrambled Words

1. deadmici ______________ (healthcare for the poor)
2. enscikis ______________ (involves body language)
3. fracitinecito ______________ (an indication of competency)
4. gloomyheat ______________ (lab area that counts blood cells)
5. irebrar ______________ (message obstruction)
6. mexicrops ______________ (involves one's concept of space)
7. ratyitre ______________ (highly complex care)
8. shymictre ______________ (most lab tests are this type)
9. sneeviconte ______________ (phlebotomy)
10. troblumaya ______________ (describes most outpatients)

KNOWLEDGE DRILL 1-3: HISTORICAL PHLEBOTOMY EVENTS

Number the following events in chronological order from 1 through 5, with 1 being the earliest recorded event.

a. ______ The French used leeching for localized bloodletting.

b. ______ "Short robe" surgeons used cupping and leeching to extract blood.

c. ______ Microsurgeons use leeching to lessen the complications of surgery.

d. ______ Hippocrates used bloodletting to cleanse the body of impurities.

e. ______ Physicians used a procedure called venesection to treat George Washington.

KNOWLEDGE DRILL 1-4: INPATIENT/OUTPATIENT FACILITY

Write the correct category (outpatient or inpatient) of healthcare facility in the line provided before the statement description.

1. ______________________ Principal source of healthcare services for most people
2. ______________________ Highly complex services
3. ______________________ Requires that patients stay overnight or longer
4. ______________________ Center of the American healthcare system
5. ______________________ Same-day surgical procedures
6. ______________________ Physician's office care

KNOWLEDGE DRILL 1-5: MEDICARE/MEDICAID PROGRAMS

Write the correct program name (Medicare or Medicaid) in the line provided before the statement description.

1. ______________________ Funds come from federal grants
2. ______________________ An entitlement program
3. ______________________ Provides medical assistance to the poor
4. ______________________ Program administered by the state
5. ______________________ Benefits divided into two sections: Part A and Part B
6. ______________________ Financed through social security deductions

KNOWLEDGE DRILL 1-6: PROFESSIONAL ATTITUDE

After each characteristic listed below, define and describe how this quality contributes to your professional attitude:

a. Self-confidence ______________________

b. Self-motivation ______________________

c. Compassion ______________________

d. Dependability ______________________

e. Ethical behavior ______________________

f. Integrity ______________________

Skills Drills

SKILLS DRILL 1-1: REQUISITION ACTIVITY

Instructions: A test requisition contains the following test abbreviations. Write the complete name of the test and the department that will perform the test on the corresponding line next to the abbreviation.

Any Hospital USA
1123 West Physician Drive
Any Town USA

Laboratory Test Requisition

PATIENT INFORMATION:

Name: Smith (last) Jane (first) R (MI)

Identification Number: 09365784 Birth Date: 06/21/63

Referring Physician: Coleman

Date to be Collected: 03/11/11 Time to be Collected: 0600

Special Instructions: line draw only

TEST(S) REQUIRED:

TEST ABBREVIATION	TEST NAME	DEPARTMENT
1. RBC	RED BLOOD CELL COUNT	CBC, HEMOGRAM
2. Hgb	HEMOGLOBIN	CBC, HEMOGRAM
3. FDP	FIBRIN SPLIT PRODUCTS	COAGULATION
4. LD	LACTATE DEHYDROGENASE	CHEMISTRY
5. PT	PROTHROMBIN TIME	COAGULATION
6. CBC	COMPLETE BLOOD COUNT	HEMOGRAM
7. CEA	CARCINOEMBRYONIC ANTIGEN	CHEMISTRY
8. RPR	RAPID PLASMA REAGIN	SEROLOGY / IMMUNOLOGY
9. UA	URINALYSIS	URINALYSIS
10. C&S	CULTURE AND SENSATIVITY	MICROBIOLOGY

SKILLS DRILL 1-2: WORD BUILDING (See Chapter 4, Medical Terminology)

Divide each of the words below into all of its elements (parts): prefix (P), word root (WR), combining vowel (CV), and suffix (S). Write the word part, its definition, and the meaning of the word on the corresponding lines. If the word does not have a particular element, write NA (not applicable) in its place.

Example: pathology

Elements ________ / *path* / *o* / *logy*
P WR CV S

Definitions ________ / *disease* / ____ / *study of*

Meaning: study of disease

1. nephrology

Elements ________ / ________ / ____ / ________
P WR CV S

Definition ________ / ________ / ____ / ________

Meaning:

2. phlebotomy

Elements ________ / ________ / ____ / ________
P WR CV S

Definition ________ / ________ / ____ / ________

Meaning:

3. polycythemia

Elements ________ / ________ / ____ / ________
P WR CV S

Definition ________ / ________ / ____ / ________

Meaning:

4. hematology

Elements ________ / ________ / ____ / ________
P WR CV S

Definition ________ / ________ / ____ / ________

Meaning:

5. erythrocyte

Elements ________ / ________ / ____ / ________
P WR CV S

Definition ________ / ________ / ____ / ________

Meaning:

6. dermatologist

Elements ________ / ________ / ____ / ________
P WR CV S

Definition ________ / ________ / ____ / ________

Meaning:

SKILLS DRILL 1-3: PROPER TELEPHONE ETIQUETTE

Fill in the blanks of the following table with the missing information.

Proper Etiquette	Communication Tips	Rationale
Answer (1) ______________.		• If the phone is allowed to ring too many times, the caller may assume that the people working in the laboratory are inefficient or (2)______________.
State your name and department.		• The caller has a right to know to whom he or she is speaking.
Be helpful.	Ask how you can be of help to (3) ______________ and facilitate the conversation. Keep your statements and answers simple and to the point so as to avoid confusion.	• When a phone rings, it is because someone needs something. Because of the nature of the healthcare business, the caller may be (4) ______________ and may benefit from hearing a calm, pleasant voice at the other end
(5) ______________ calls.	Inform a caller whose call is interrupting one from someone else. Always ask permission before putting a caller on hold in case it is an (6) _________ that must be handled immediately	• It takes an organized person to coordinate several calls. • The caller should be informed if he or she is interrupting another call.
Transfer and (7) ______________ ______________.	Tell a caller when you are going to transfer the call or put it on hold and learn how to do this properly. **Note:** Do not leave the line open and do not keep the caller waiting too long.	• Disconnecting callers while transferring or putting them on hold (8) ______________________. • Leaving the line open so that other conversations can be heard by the person on hold is discourteous and can compromise (9) ________________. • (10) ________________ with a caller when on hold for longer than expected; this keeps him or her informed of the circumstance. • If a caller is waiting on hold too long, ask if he or she would like to leave a message.
Be prepared to record information.	Have a pencil and paper close to the phone. (11) __________________, which means clarifying, (12) __________, and summarizing the information received.	• Documentation is necessary when answering the phone at work to ensure that (13)______________ information is transmitted to the necessary person. • Reading back the information when complete is one of best ways to (14)__________ it is correct.

Proper Etiquette	Communication Tips	Rationale
Know the laboratory's policies.	Make answers consistent by learning the laboratory's policies.	• People who answer the telephone must know the (15) ______________ to avoid giving the wrong information. • (16) ______________ help establish the laboratory's credibility, because a caller's perception of the lab involves more than just accurate test results.
Defuse (17) ____________ situations.	When a caller is hostile, you might say "I can see why you are upset. Let me see what I can do."	• Some callers become angry because of lost results or errors in billing. • (18) ____________ a hostile caller's (19) __________ will often defuse the situation. • After the caller has calmed down, the issue can be addressed.
Try to assist everyone.	If you are uncertain, refer the caller to someone who can address the caller's issue. Remind yourself to keep your attention on (23) __________ ____________ at a time.	• It is possible to assist callers and (20) ____________ __________ even if you are not actually answering their questions. • Validate callers' requests by giving a response that tells them (21) ______________________. • (22) ________________ in the caller will enhance communication and contribute to the good (24) ____________ of the laboratory.

SKILLS DRILL 1-4: TWO CATEGORIES OF HEALTHCARE FACILITIES

Outpatient

- (1) ______________ of healthcare services for most people.
- Offer (3) ____________ care in physician's office to (4) ______________ care in a freestanding ambulatory setting.
- Serve (5) ______________ physicians who assume (7) ____________ responsibility for maintaining patients' health.
- Serve (8) ______________ physicians (specialists) who perform routine surgery, (10) ______________ treatments, therapeutic radiology, and so on in same-day service centers.

Inpatient

- The key resource and (2) ___________ of the American healthcare system.
- Offer specialized instrumentation and technology to assist in unusual diagnoses and treatments.
- Serve (6) _____________ (highly complex services and therapy) practitioners. Usually requires that patients stay overnight or longer.
- Examples are acute care hospitals, nursing homes, (9) _____________, hospices, and rehabilitation centers.

Crossword

ACROSS

1. Federal healthcare program for persons 65 years of age and older
6. Occupational Safety & Health Administration (abbrev.)
8. Personalized filters or biases
10. Internationally recognized standard formula for PT results
11. Electroencephalogram (abbrev.)
12. Protected health information (abbrev.)
14. State of being varied or different
17. Cervical smear for cancer cells
18. Complete blood counts (abbrev.)
19. Continuing education unit (abbrev.)
20. Center for Medicare and Medicaid (abbrev.)
22. Identifying with the feelings of another person
23. Therapeutic nonverbal communication
27. Disseminated intravascular coagulation (abbrev.)
29. Intensive care unit
31. Cardiac marker test used in the ER
33. Arizona's version of Medicaid
35. Gamma-glutamyl transferase (abbrev.)
36. Testing of urine (abbrev.)
37. "Blood ________" to rid body of evil spirits
39. Health maintenance organization (abbrev.)
40. Word meaning "immediate"
42. Emotion brought on by feeling out of control
43. Alanine aminotransferase (abbrev.)

DOWN

1. Hemoglobin concentration in RBCs (abbrev.)
2. Standard or requirement for a technical specialty
3. Registered nurses (abbrev.)
4. Wrongful act committed against one's person
5. Study of nonverbal communication
7. Decrease in number of RBCs in blood
8. Cardiac marker test used in the ER
9. Standards of right or wrong conduct
13. Federal HC program for the indigent
15. Unquestioning belief in the HCW's ability
16. ________ stain for bacteria
21. American Hospital Association (abbrev.)
22. Complete removal of all blood
24. Occupation therapy (abbrev.)
25. Organization that offers continuing education
26. Federal law that protects patient confidentiality
28. Personal standard of honesty
30. __________ *medicinalis*
32. Testing at the point of care (abbrev.)
34. To confirm specific qualifications have been met
37. Laboratory information system (abbrev.)
38. One of the national phlebotomy certifying agencies
39. Hematocrit
41. Turnaround time (abbrev.)

Chapter Review Questions

1. In the 17th century, the name given to the bloodletting tool or lancet was:
   a. cup.
   b. fleam.
   c. hemostat.
   d. leech.

2. A factor that contributes to the overall professional impression made by the phlebotomist is:
   a. compassion.
   b. dependability.
   c. self-confidence.
   d. any of the above.

3. After successful completion of the American Medical Technologists phlebotomy examination, the initials for the title granted are:
   a. CPT.
   b. CLT.
   c. PBT.
   d. RPT.

4. Understanding the ____________ of a diverse population is very important in providing healthcare.
   a. ethics
   b. history
   c. motivation
   d. traditions

5. The evidence that an individual has mastered fundamental competencies in his or her technical area is called:
   a. certification.
   b. ethics.
   c. esteem.
   d. tort.

6. An example of a type of coding for diagnoses is:
   a. CLIA.
   b. DRG.
   c. Medicare.
   d. OSHA.

7. Which of the following is the responsibility of a phlebotomist?
   a. Analyze specimens
   b. Collect drug screens
   c. Obtain vital signs
   d. Transport patients

8. Which of the following is an example of proxemics?
   a. Eye contact
   b. Zone of comfort
   c. Facial expressions
   d. Personal hygiene

9. Which of the following is improper telephone technique?
   a. Listening and restating information
   b. Putting an irritated caller on hold
   c. Taking notes as the caller is talking
   d. Referring the caller elsewhere if uncertain

10. A healthcare facility that provides ambulatory services is:
    a. an acute-care hospital.
    b. a nursing home.
    c. a rehabilitation center.
    d. an urgent care center.

11. The name of a federal entitlement program is
    a. IDS.
    b. HIPPA.
    c. managed care.
    d. Medicare.

12. The specialty that treats disorders of the brain is called:
    a. cardiology.
    b. gerontology.
    c. neurology.
    d. pathology.

13. The department in the hospital that treats lung deficiencies is:
    a. the clinical laboratory.
    b. diagnostic imaging.
    c. electroneurodiagnostics.
    d. respiratory therapy.

14. The histology department in the laboratory performs:
    a. blood culture testing.
    b. compatibility testing.
    c. electrolyte monitoring.
    d. tissue processing.

15. The abbreviation for the routine chemistry test that detects colorectal cancer is called:
    a. BUN.
    b. CEA.
    c. GTT.
    d. LD.

16. Which of the following laboratory professionals is specified by CLIA'88 as responsible for evaluating new procedures?
    a. Laboratory manager
    b. Medical laboratory scientist
    c. Medical laboratory technician
    d. Technical supervisor

CASE STUDIES

Case Study 1-1: More Education for the OJT Phlebotomist

The phlebotomist, Sam, has been trained OJT, and since that is how everyone else currently in the physician's office was trained, he doesn't see it as a problem. One thing bothers him, however, and it is that no one seems to be able to answer questions that come up daily about the rationale for doing phlebotomy procedures a certain way. The answer is always the same: "I don't know. It has always been done that way." When the physician's office was notified of a pending visit from CLIA inspectors, it was decided that all the phlebotomists should get credentials, if possible, and in that way every phlebotomist would better understand his or her job responsibilities.

QUESTIONS

1. What does "getting credentialed" mean as far as phlebotomists are concerned?
2. How can Sam become officially recognized as a phlebotomist?
3. Where can Sam go to receive a standardized educational curriculum that incorporates classroom instruction and clinical practice in phlebotomy?
4. How can Sam keep current after he becomes credentialed?

Case Study 1-2: Nonverbal Cues Speak Loudly

The patient did not understand English, but this was not unusual in the County Hospital. Donna, the phlebotomist, spoke only English and could not tell the patient why she was there or what was going to happen. She had learned that the best way to handle this situation was to continue preparing her equipment, nodding her head often to affirm the patient's comments, but never really looking the patient in the eye. This particular time the patient continued to talk nervously and did not offer his arm. As Donna glanced up to see why he hadn't, she saw an intense frown on his face and that his eyes were narrowed. His hand was actually clenched and he was leaning back in his bed as far as he could. Donna proceeded by grasping his arm and forcefully moving it toward her. She quickly tied the tourniquet, cleaned the area, and prepared to stick the median cubital vein. Just as she got the needle through the skin, the patient yelled and pulled the needle out of his arm.

QUESTIONS

1. What did Donna's nonverbal cues say to the patient?
2. What nonverbal signals was the patient offering to Donna?
3. What should the facial and hand cues from the patient have told Donna?
4. How could this situation have been handled differently?

CHAPTER

2

Quality Assurance and Legal Issues

OBJECTIVES

Study the information in your textbook that corresponds to each objective to prepare yourself for the activities in this chapter.

1. Define the key terms and abbreviations listed at the beginning of this chapter.
2. Identify national organizations, agencies, and regulations that support quality assurance in healthcare.
3. Define quality improvement and identify ways that it can be implemented in HC organizations.
4. List and describe the components of a quality assurance (QA) program and identify areas in phlebotomy subject to QC.
5. Demonstrate knowledge of the legal aspects associated with phlebotomy procedures and describe situations that may have legal ramifications.
6. Define legal terminology associated with healthcare settings and describe how a phlebotomist can avoid litigation.

Matching

Use choices only once unless otherwise indicated.

MATCHING 2-1: KEY TERMS AND DESCRIPTIONS

Match the key term with the *best* description.

Key Terms (1–15)

1. ______ Assault
2. ______ Battery
3. ______ Breach of confidentiality
4. ______ Civil action
5. ______ CLSI
6. ______ CMS
7. ______ CQI
8. ______ Defendant
9. ______ Delta check
10. ______ Deposition
11. ______ Discovery
12. ______ Due care
13. ______ Fraud
14. ______ GLPs
15. ______ Informed consent

Descriptions

A. Act or threat causing another to be in fear of immediate battery
B. Federal agency that administers the CLIA
C. Organization that develops voluntary standards and guidelines for the laboratory
D. Compares current lab test results with previous results for the same test on the same patient
E. Deceitful practice or false portrayal of facts either by words or by conduct
F. Program designed to nationally standardize measurements of performance
G. Failure to keep privileged medical information private
H. Formal process in litigation that involves taking depositions and interrogating parties involved
I. Practices that emphasize quality assurance when in any laboratory setting
J. Implies voluntary and competent permission for a medical procedure, test, or medication
K. Intentional offensive touching or use of force without consent or legal justification
L. Legal actions in which the alleged injured party sues for monetary damages
M. Level of care a person with good sense provides under given circumstances
N. Person against whom a complaint is filed
O. When one party questions another under oath with a court reporter present

Match the key term with the *best* description.

Key Terms (16–30)

16. ______ Invasion of privacy
17. ______ Malpractice
18. ______ Negligence
19. ______ NPSGs
20. ______ Plaintiff
21. ______ QA
22. ______ QC
23. ______ QSE
24. ______ Quality indicators
25. ______ *Respondeat superior*
26. ______ Standard of care
27. ______ Statute of limitations
28. ______ Threshold values
29. ______ Tort
30. ______ Vicarious liability

Descriptions

A. Failure to exercise due care
B. Guides used to monitor all areas of patient care
C. Injured party in the litigation process
D. Latin phrase meaning "let the master respond"
E. Length of time after alleged injury in which a lawsuit can be filed
F. Level of acceptable practice beyond which quality care cannot be assured
G. Liability imposed on one person for acts committed by another
H. Level of care and skill that provides due care for patients
I. Overall process that established policies and procedures for assured quality
J. A component of a CQI program that is a form of procedural control
K. Safety practices for protecting patients and advancing quality care
L. A core set of systems essentials for quality outcomes
M. Type of negligence implying a greater standard of care was owed to the injured person
N. Violation of one's right to be left alone
O. Wrongful act committed against one's person, property, or reputation

MATCHING 2-2: TYPE OF CONSENT

Type of Consent

1. ______ Informed consent
2. ______ Expressed consent
3. ______ Implied consent
4. ______ HIV consent
5. ______ Minor consent
6. ______ Refusal of consent

Description

a. A constitutional right to refuse a medical procedure
b. Consent is implied by actions
c. Implies voluntary and competent permission
d. Parental/guardian consent required for medical treatment
e. Required before surgery or high-risk procedures
f. State laws specify what type of information must be given

MATCHING 2-3: STEPS IN WORKFLOW PATH AND INDICATORS

Match the indicators that monitor quality service to the appropriate step in the workflow path.

Indicators

1. ______ Duplicate test ordering
2. ______ Accuracy of ordering
3. ______ Wristband evaluation
4. ______ Transit time
5. ______ Employee retention
6. ______ Sample acceptability
7. ______ Safety
8. ______ Self-assessments

Step in Workflow Path

A. Process control
B. Specimen transport
C. Internal assessment
D. Patient assessment
E. Specimen receiving/processing
F. Specimen collection/labeling
G. Test request
H. Personnel

Labeling Exercises

LABELING 2-1: MICROBIOLOGY QUALITY ASSESSMENT FORM (Text Fig. 2-1)

Answers to the following questions can be found on the Quality Assessment and Improvement Tracking form below. Circle the answer on the form; write the number of the question in or near the circle; then write out the answer on the appropriate line.

HOSPITAL & HEALTH CENTER

QUALITY ASSESSMENT AND IMPROVEMENT TRACKING

CONFIDENTIAL A.R.S. 36-445 et. seq.

STANDARD OF CARE/SERVICE:

IMPORTANT ASPECT OF CARE/SERVICE:
LABORATORY SERVICES
COLLECTION/TRANSPORT

SIGNATURES:

DIRECTOR

MEDICAL DIRECTOR

VICE PRESIDENT/ADMINISTRATOR

DEPARTMENTS:
DATA SOURCE(S):
METHODOLOGY: [X] RETROSPECTIVE [ ] CONCURRENT
TYPE: [ ] STRUCTURE [ ] PROCESS [X] OUTCOME
PERSON RESPONSIBLE FOR:
- DATA COLLECTION: J. HERRIG
- DATA ORGANIZATION: J. HERRIG
- ACTION PLAN: J. HERRIG
- FOLLOW-UP: J. HERRIG

DATE MONITORING BEGAN: 1990
TIME PERIOD THIS MONITOR: 2ND QUARTER 2009
MONITOR DISCONTINUED BECAUSE:
FOLLOW-UP:

INDICATORS	THLD	ACT	PREV	CRITICAL ANALYSIS/EVALUATION	ACTION PLAN
Blood Culture contamination rate will not exceed 3%				Population: All patients All monthly indicators were under threshold, 3%	Share results and analysis with Lab staff and ER staff.
APR - # of Draws: 713 # Contaminated: 13	3.00%	1.8%	1.2%	% Contamination from draws other than Line draws, by unit:	
MAY - # of Draws: 710 # Contaminated: 23	3.00%	2.8%	2.3%	APR: ER = 4.7% Lab = 0.7% MAY: ER = 11.5% Lab = 1.0% JUN: ER = 8.6% Lab = 1.1%	
JUN - # of Draws: 702 # Contaminated: 17	3.00%	2.4%	1.9%	ER was over threshold for each month of quarter.	
Total for 1st Quarter - # of Draws: 2125 # Contaminated: 50	3.00%	2.4%	1.9%		

1. What is being used by the Microbiology Department as a blood culture quality indicator? CONTAIMANATION RATE NOT TO EXCEED 3%
2. What is the acceptable threshold? 3%
3. What was the actual percentage contamination for the first quarter? 2.4%
4. What month has the highest contamination from ER draws? MAY 11.5%
5. What was the rate of contamination by the lab in the same month? 1.0%
6. What is the action plan for blood culture QA? SHARE RESULTS WITH ER & LAB

LABELING 2-2: NURSING SERVICES MANUAL

Identify each numbered item on this portion of Nursing Service Manual (text Fig. 2-2) and write the answer on the corresponding numbered line below.

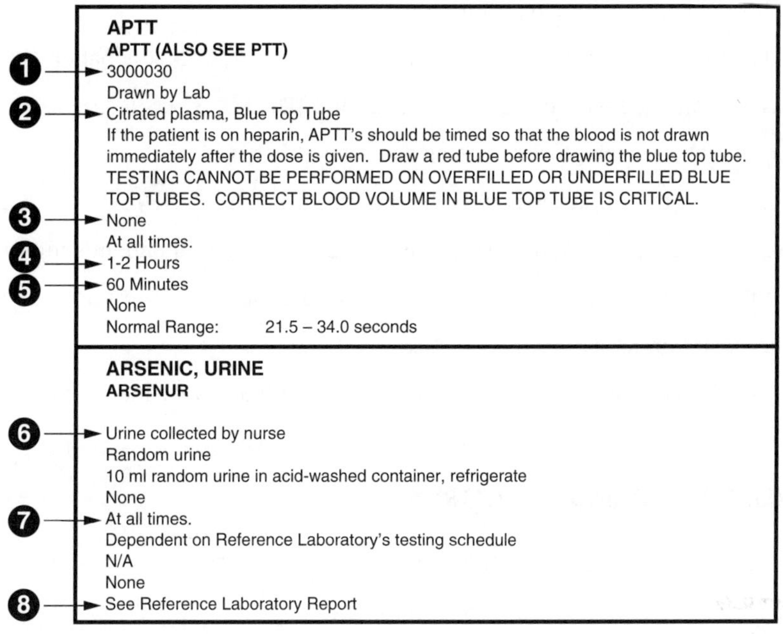
APTT
APTT (ALSO SEE PTT)
3000030
Drawn by Lab
Citrated plasma, Blue Top Tube
If the patient is on heparin, APTT's should be timed so that the blood is not drawn immediately after the dose is given. Draw a red tube before drawing the blue top tube. TESTING CANNOT BE PERFORMED ON OVERFILLED OR UNDERFILLED BLUE TOP TUBES. CORRECT BLOOD VOLUME IN BLUE TOP TUBE IS CRITICAL.
None
At all times.
1-2 Hours
60 Minutes
None
Normal Range: 21.5 – 34.0 seconds

ARSENIC, URINE
ARSENUR
Urine collected by nurse
Random urine
10 ml random urine in acid-washed container, refrigerate
None
At all times.
Dependent on Reference Laboratory's testing schedule
N/A
None
See Reference Laboratory Report

1. ______________________________
2. ______________________________
3. ______________________________
4. ______________________________
5. ______________________________
6. ______________________________
7. ______________________________
8. ______________________________

Knowledge Drills

KNOWLEDGE DRILL 2-1: CAUTIONS AND KEY POINT RECOGNITION

The following sentences are taken from "Caution" statements found throughout the Chapter 2 text. Using the TEXTBOOK, fill in the blanks with the missing information.

1. A phlebotomist who attempts to collect a blood specimen (A) ____________ the patient's (B) ____________ can be charged with (C) ____________ and (D) ____________.
2. If a neglectful act occurs while an employee is doing something that is (A) ____________ within his or her duties or (B) ____________, the employee may be held (C) ____________ (D) ____________ for that act.
3. A hospital, as an (A) ____________, cannot escape (B) ____________ for a patient's injury simply by (C) ____________ out various services to other persons and claiming it is not responsible because the party that caused the injury is not on its (D) ____________.
4. If a phlebotomist tells a patient that he or she is going to collect a blood specimen, and the patient (A) ____________ out an arm, it is considered (B) ____________ (C) ____________.

KNOWLEDGE DRILL 2-2: SCRAMBLED WORDS

Aedtl DELTA (a quality check)

Drisotacin INDICATORS (used to monitor QA)

Fatpiflin PLAINTIFF (an injured party)

Gingeencel NEGLIGENCE (not an issue if you are reasonable)

Hedlsorth THRESHOLD (exceeding this is not good)

Laquity QUALITY (must be assured in healthcare)

Savoriciu VACARIOUS (a kind of liability)

Talycodinfeitin CONFIDENTIALTY (privacy)

Ulastas ASSULT (a harmful touch)

Yencopomec COMPETENCY (an educational standard)

KNOWLEDGE DRILL 2-3: NATIONAL AGENCIES AND REGULATIONS

The following table identifies by name and abbreviation and summarizes the description, purpose, and functions of agencies and regulations described in Chapter 2 of the textbook. Using the TEXTBOOK, fill in the blanks with the missing information.

Agency/Regulation Name/Abbreviation	Description	Purpose	Functions
1. Joint (A) ______ on (B) ______ of Healthcare Organizations	A voluntary, (C) ______ agency.	Establish (D) ______ for the operation of hospitals and other health-related facilities and services	Key player in bringing (E) ______ ______ review techniques to healthcare • Largest healthcare (F) ______ ______ body in the world • Accredits over (G) ______ health care organizations
2. (A) ______ of American (B) ______	National organization whose entire membership is composed of board-certified (C) ______	Influence quality improvement in pathology and laboratory services including phlebotomy through set (D) ______ and laboratory inspection	• Offers (E) ______ ______ • Offers continuous form of laboratory (F) ______ by a team of pathologists and laboratory managers
3. (A) ______ and Laboratory (B) ______ Institute	A (C) ______, nonprofit, organization composed of representatives from the profession, industry, and government	Use a consensus process to develop (D) ______ guidelines and standards for all areas of the laboratory	• Provides guidelines and standards on which (E) ______ exam questions, program approval, and (F) ______ ______ are based

4. (A) __________ Laboratory (B) __________ Amendments of 1988	Federal regulations administered by (C) __________ that establish quality standards for all facilities that test (D) __________ specimens for the purpose of providing information used to diagnose, prevent, or treat disease or assess health status	To ensure the (E) __________, reliability, and timeliness of patient test results, regardless of the (F) __________, type or size of the laboratory	• Addresses (G) __________ assurance, quality control, proficiency testing, lab records, and personnel qualifications • Requires moderate and complex laboratory facilities to have routine inspections • Requires (H) __________ protocols for all laboratory procedures
5. (A) __________ (B) __________ Agency for Clinical Laboratory Sciences	An autonomous, nonprofit organization that is a recognized authority on (C) __________ quality	Provides accreditation or (D) __________ for clinical laboratory education programs	Provides external (E) __________ review of programs to decide if they meet certain established educational standards • Requires that phlebotomy programs meet educational standards called (F) __________

KNOWLEDGE DRILL 2-4: CRIMINAL AND CIVIL ACTIONS

On the line provided, write the correct type of legal action (civil or criminal) associated with the descriptive statement.

1. ________ Punishable by fines and/or imprisonment
2. ________ Individual may be charged with a felony or a misdemeanor
3. ________ Involves injurious acts by others in society
4. ________ Concerned with actions between two private parties
5. ________ Monetary penalties awarded in a court of law
6. ________ Constitutes the bulk of legal actions dealt with in healthcare

KNOWLEDGE DRILL 2-5: THE LITIGATION PROCESS

Number the following phases in the litigation process in chronological order from 1 through 7.

A. 5 A deposition is taken

B. 7 Appeal is filed by the losing party

C. 3 Attorney decides whether to take case or not

D. 4 Attorney files a complaint

E. 2 Injured party consults an attorney

F. 1 Patient becomes aware of prior possible injury

G. 6 Trial phase with judge and jury

KNOWLEDGE DRILL 2-6: GUIDELINES TO AVOID LAWSUITS

The following are statements concerning ways to avoid lawsuits. Finish each statement with the missing information from the TEXTBOOK.

1. Acquire informed consent VOLUNTARY AND COMPETENT PERMISSION FOR MEDICAL PROCEDURE
2. Respect a patient's RIGHT TO CONFIDENTIALITY
3. Strictly adhere to ACCEPTED PROCEDURES AND PRACTICES
4. Use proper safety CONTAINERS + DEVICES
5. Listen and respond appropriately to the PATIENTS REQUEST
6. Accurately and legibly RECORD ALL INFORMATION CONCERNING PATIENTS
7. Document INCIDENTS + OCCURENCIES
8. Perform at the prevailing STANDARD OF CARE
9. Never perform procedures that you are not TRAINED TO DO
10. Participate in continuing education to TO MAINTAIN PROFICENTCY.

Skills Drills

SKILLS DRILL 2-1: REQUISITION ACTIVITY

Instructions: Answer the following questions concerning the test requisition shown below.

1. A new phlebotomist does not know anything about collecting a D-dimer or an HIV test. Where is collection information on these tests found? IN THE SPECIMEN COLLECTION MANUAL / REQUISITION
2. What does patient consent involve when drawing an HIV sample?
   THE PROCEDURE AND WHAT IS GOING TO BE DONE.

Any Hospital USA
1123 West Physician Drive
Any Town USA

Laboratory Test Requisition

PATIENT INFORMATION:

Name: Smith (last) John (first) (MI)

Identification Number: 09365784 Birth Date: 06/21/63

Referring Physician: Payne

Date to be Collected: 03/15/11 Time to be Collected: 0600

Special Instructions: line draw only

TEST(S) REQUIRED:

____	NH4 – Ammonia	____	Gluc – glucose
____	Bili – Bilirubin, total & direct	____	Hgb – hemoglobin
____	BMP – basic metabolic panel	____	Lact – lactic acid/lactate
____	BUN – Blood urea nitrogen	____	Plt. Ct. – platelet count
____	Lytes – electrolytes	____	PT – prothrombin time
____	CBC – complete blood count	____	PTT – partial thromboplastin time
____	Chol – cholesterol	____	RPR – rapid plasma regain
____	ESR – erythrocyte sed rate	____	T&S – type and screen
____	EtOH – alcohol	____	PSA – prostatic specific antigen
X	D-dimer	Other	HIV

SKILLS DRILL 2-2: WORD BUILDING

Divide each of the words below into all of its elements (parts): prefix (P), word root (WR), combining vowel (CV), and suffix (S). Write the word part, its definition, and the meaning of the word on the corresponding lines. If the word does not have a particular element, write NA (not applicable) in its place.

Example: pathologists

Elements ______ / *path* / *o* / *logists*
P WR CV S

Definitions ______ / *disease* / ______ / *specialist in the study of*

Meaning: a specialist who studies and interprets disease

1. Tachometer

Elements ______ / ______ / ______ / ______
P WR CV S

Definitions ______ / ______ / ______ / ______

Meaning:

2. Phlebotomy

Elements ______ / ______ / ______ / ______
P WR CV S

Definitions ______ / ______ / ______ / ______

Meaning:

3. Postanalytical

Elements ______ / ______ / ______ / ______
P WR CV S

Definitions ______ / ______ / ______ / ______

Meaning:

4. Chronology

Elements ______ / ______ / ______ / ______
P WR CV S

Definitions ______ / ______ / ______ / ______

Meaning:

SKILLS DRILL 2-3: CLIA WEB SITE

Go to the Centers for Medicare and Medicaid Services Web site. Find the section on Regulations and Guidance. Find information about CLIA in the section on Legislation. Find a link to information regarding Certificate of Waiver Laboratory Project. Look for the pdf file entitled Good Laboratory Practices. Use the glossary in that document to answer the following questions in the spaces provided.

1. Define the following terms:

   a. Medwatch ______________________________

   ____

   ____

   b. Pipet ______________________________

   ____

   ____

   c. Reagent ______________________________

   ____

   ____

   d. Package insert ______________________________

   ____

   ____

2. Identify the last tube to be collected under the glossary entry "routine order of draw." ______________________________

   ____

3. How many questions are to be asked in a laboratory's self-examination according to the QA glossary entry?

   ____

SKILLS DRILL 2-4: AMERICAN HOSPITAL ASSOCIATION WEB SITE

A. Go to the American Hospital Association's Web site (AHA. org). Find the Resource Center. Find the pull-down menu entitled "Issues." Scroll down to the "Quality and Patient Safety" listing.

1. Write the first sentence of the beginning paragraph on the lines that follow: ______________________________

____

2. Click on "Hospitals in Pursuit of Excellence"; choose "Patient Safety" from the listed resources. Click on "View Full Summary" at the end of the article. What are the deaths annually attributed to medical errors as stated in article entitled "To Err is Human: Building a Safer Health System"? ______________________________

____

3. Name an organization listed in the summary that is playing a major role in advancing safe practices through its Patient Safety Goals that are updated annually, ______________________________

____

____

4. From the listing "Serious Adverse Events," choose "Health Care-Acquired Infections" and record how much money is estimated being spent yearly on healthcare-associated infections. ______________________________

____

B. Go to the American Hospital Association's Web site. Find the Resource Center. Choose the "About" pull-down menu and click on "Patient Care Partnership." Read the preferred language version of the Patient Care Partnership brochure and answer the following questions in the space provided.

1. State the name of the notice in the brochure under "Protection of Your Privacy" that describes to the patients how they can get a copy of information from records about their care. ______________________________

____

2. Under "Preparing you and your family for when you leave the hospital," find a statement that talks about follow-up care.

____

Crossword

ACROSS

1. A type of negligence
3. Black stripes corresponding to letters and numbers
5. Person against whom the complaint is filed
8. Information collected for analysis
10. Clinical and Laboratory Sciences Institute
11. The state of being liable
12. Quality assurance (abbrev.)
13. Injured party
17. Complete test package
19. Where 10% of malpractice lawsuits end up
20. Complete medical file of a patient is called a ________
21. Level of normal care, ____ care
22. Common abbrev. for physicians' title (pl)
24. Anyone who has not reached age of minority
25. Begins legal proceedings
26. To give permission for medical procedure
27. Agency that manages federal HC programs (abbrev.)
28. Failure to observe a law or promise
30. Type of legal action in which the party sues for monetary damages
34. National agency that accredits lab programs
36. _______ control or assurance
37. Judge the worth of

DOWN

1. Provides healthcare to person over 65 years of age
2. Number of QA recommendations for COWs
4. Federal rules and regulations for all diagnostic labs
6. Check that compares current results with previous ones
7. Turnaround time
9. Trace by means of evidence
13. Lawyers are said to ________ law
14. Events or minor conflicts
15. Realities or truths
16. Hurt, damage, or injury
18. General course or drift (pl)
21. Taking deposition and interrogating persons
23. Another abbrev. for SGOT
28. Hematoma/injury and discoloring of skin
29. Intentional threat of immediate harm
31. Based on the law
32. Use of checks and controls (abbrev.)
33. Deceitful practice
35. Chance of injury, damage, or loss

Chapter Review Questions

1. This organization establishes standards for the operation of hospitals and other healthcare facilities and services.
   a. American Hospital Association
   b. College of American Pathology
   c. National Accrediting Agency
   d. The Joint Commission

2. An agency that manages the federal healthcare programs of Medicare and Medicaid is the:
   a. CAP.
   b. CLIA.
   c. CLSI.
   d. CMS.

3. This is an early warning policy to help healthcare organizations identify unfavorable actions and takes step to prevent them.
   a. Quality indicators
   b. Quality Systems Essentials
   c. Sentinel events
   d. Thresholds values

4. These measurable, objective guides are established to monitor all aspects of patient care.
   a. Indicators
   b. Outcomes
   c. Procedures
   d. Threshold values

5. Which manual describes the chemical, electrical, and radiation safety for the laboratory?
   a. Collection manual
   b. Infection control manual
   c. Procedure manual
   d. Safety manual

6. One of the generic steps in risk management is
   a. assessment of work patterns.
   b. education of the employees.
   c. evaluation of medical records.
   d. review of employees' records.

7. Informed consent means that:
   a. a patient's medical records are available for review by all healthcare workers.
   b. all consequences of a medical procedure have been given to the patient.
   c. the patient received a book outlining all procedures and their consequences.
   d. the patient's confidentiality has been breached during the assessment process.

8. This is a national organization that develops guidelines and sets standards for laboratory procedures.
   a. CAP
   b. CLIAC
   c. CLSI
   d. NAACLS

9. A phlebotomist hired by a hospital as a temporary employee commits a negligent act for which the hospital is liable. This is an example of:
   a. assault and battery.
   b. *res ipsa loquitur.*
   c. respondeat superior.
   d. standard of care.

10. A phlebotomist collects a sample from a 16-year-old patient without obtaining parental or guardian consent. Which of the following could the phlebotomist be charged with?
    a. assault and battery
    b. invasion of privacy
    c. statute of limitations
    d. vicarious liability

11. National Patient Safety Goals (NPSGs) are:
    a. rules set down by CDC and overseen by OSHA.
    b. standards set by NAACLS for educational programs.
    c. the Joint Commission's specific safety requirements.
    d. voluntary guidelines and protocol written by CLSI.

12. A comparison of current test results with previous results for the same test on the same patient is called a:
    a. delta check.
    b. quality indicator.
    c. quality system essential.
    d. sentinel event.

13. Which one of the following forms states the concern and describes the corrective action when a problem occurs?
    a. Equipment check form
    b. Delta review form
    c. Internal report
    d. Quality control check

14. A type of negligence committed by a professional is called:
    a. assault.
    b. battery.
    c. invasion of privacy.
    d. malpractice.

15. Failure to keep privileged medical information private is:
    a. breach of confidentiality.
    b. invasion of privacy.
    c. *res ipsa loquitur.*
    d. vicarious liability.

CASE STUDIES

Case Study 2-1: Quality Assurance in a COW Laboratory

The COW lab in a large internal medicine group practice performed over 50 waived tests a day. The medical assistants and the phlebotomists who performed the waived testing were all trained OJTs. It was obvious from the inconsistent results recorded on the cumulative report that everyone's technique differed somewhat. When notification came from CLIA that they would be visiting the site within the next month, the lead physician decided that a QA process had to be put into place. He directed the lab staff to the CLIA Web site for instructions on waived testing standardization in the form of GLPs issued by CLIAC.

QUESTIONS

1. What are CLIA and CLIAC?
2. Why is CLIA visiting their site?
3. What are the GLPs and what makes them valuable in standardizing the waived testing process?
4. What are other examples of QC components that could be put in place in this lab setting?

Case Study 2-2: Blood Draw Fails Delta Check

It was a very busy day in the hospital laboratory since two phlebotomists were out for medical reasons. An order came from the fourth floor for a timed draw. Joe, a phlebotomist from a temporary agency, was still there, even though he was supposed to have gotten off 2 hours earlier. No one was there to collect the specimen except Joe. Knowing how important it was, he decided to go ahead and collect it. When he arrived in the room, the patient was seated in a chair between the beds. Joe asked the patient his name and in which bed he belonged. When the seated patient answered with the right last name and pointed to the correct bed, Joe proceeded to collect the specimen from him while he sat in the chair. Joe labeled the specimen tubes at the nursing station while noting the draw on the desk clipboard. When a second specimen was drawn from the patient later that morning, it failed the delta check. The second specimen was recollected and the results showed the specimen that Joe had drawn to be in error.

QUESTIONS

1. What is a delta check?
2. What do you see that could have caused this discrepancy?
3. What should Joe have done differently?
4. What were Joe's obligations to the laboratory after his regular shift?
5. Who is ultimately responsible for Joe's actions while he is at work?

CHAPTER

3

Infection Control, Safety, First Aid, and Personal Wellness

OBJECTIVES

Study the information in the textbook that corresponds to each objective to prepare yourself for the activities in this chapter.

1. Define the key terms and abbreviations listed at the beginning of this chapter.
2. Identify the components of the chain of infection and give examples of each, describe infection-control procedures used to break the chain, and identify four functions of infection-control programs.
3. Describe proper procedures for hand hygiene, putting on and removing protective clothing, and entering the nursery or neonatal ICU.
4. Describe standard and transmission-based precautions and identify the organizations that developed them.
5. State safety rules to follow when working in the laboratory and in patient areas.
6. List examples of blood-borne pathogens and describe their means of transmission in a healthcare setting.
7. Discuss the major points of the Bloodborne Pathogens (BBP) Standard, including changes required by the Needlestick Safety and Prevention Act, and identify key elements of a BBP exposure-control plan.
8. Describe hazards, identify warning symbols, list actions to take if incidents occur, and specify rules to follow for proper biologic, electrical, fire, radiation, and chemical safety.
9. Identify symptoms of shock, state first aid procedures for treating external hemorrhage and shock, identify the main points of the International CPR and ECC guidelines, and identify the links in the **American Heart Association Chain of Survival.**
10. Describe the role of personal hygiene, proper nutrition, rest, exercise, back protection, and stress management in personal wellness.

Matching

Use choices only once unless otherwise indicated.

MATCHING 3-1: KEY TERMS AND DESCRIPTIONS

Match each key term with the *best* description.

Key Terms (1–19)

1. ____ BBP
2. ____ biohazard
3. ____ CDC
4. ____ chain of infection
5. ____ engineering controls
6. ____ EPA
7. ____ fire tetrahedron
8. ____ fomites
9. ____ HAI
10. ____ HazCom
11. ____ HBV
12. ____ HCV
13. ____ HICPAC
14. ____ HIV
15. ____ immune
16. ____ infectious/causative agent
17. ____ isolation procedures
18. ____ microbe
19. ____ MSDS

Descriptions (1–19)

A. A series of components or events that lead to an infection
B. Anything harmful or potentially harmful to health
C. Chemistry of fire representation
D. Devices that isolate or remove a workplace BBP hazard
E. Contains general, precautionary, and emergency information for a hazardous product
F. Federal agency charged with the investigation and control of certain diseases
G. Federal agency that regulates the disposal of hazardous waste
H. Federal organization that advises the CDC on nosocomial infection prevention guidelines
I. Hepatitis B virus
J. Hepatitis C virus
K. Inanimate objects that can harbor material containing infectious agents
L. Infection associated with a healthcare facility
M. OSHA standard requiring employers to maintain documentation on hazardous chemicals
N. Pathogen responsible for causing an infection
O. Procedures that separate patients with certain transmissible infections from others
P. Protected from or resistant to a particular disease or infection
Q. Short for microorganism
R. Term applied to infectious microorganisms in blood and other body fluids
S. Virus that causes acquired immunodeficiency syndrome (AIDS)

Key Terms (20–37)

20. ____ neutropenic
21. ____ NIOSH
22. ____ nosocomial infection
23. ____ OSHA
24. ____ parenteral
25. ____ pathogenic
26. ____ pathogens
27. ____ percutaneous
28. ____ permucosal
29. ____ PPE
30. ____ reservoir
31. ____ reverse isolation
32. ____ standard precautions

Descriptions (20–37)

A. Any route other than the digestive tract.
B. Capable of causing disease
C. Federal agency that recommends ways to prevent work-related injury
D. Federal agency that mandates and enforces safe working conditions for employees
E. Having an abnormally low neutrophil count
F. Individual who has little resistance to an infectious agent.
G. Infection acquired in a hospital
H. Microorganisms capable of causing disease
I. Practices that alter how tasks are performed to reduce the likelihood of BBP exposure
J. Precautions that reduce the risk of airborne, droplet, or contact transmission
K. Precautions to be used in caring for all patients
L. Protects a patient who is highly susceptible to infection
M. Protective items worn by an individual
N. Source of an infectious microorganism
O. Through mucous membranes
P. Through the skin

33. ____ susceptible host

34. ____ transmission-based precautions

35. ____ vector transmission

36. ____ vehicle transmission

37. ____ work practice controls

Q. Transmission of an infectious agent by an insect, arthropod, or animal

R. Transmission of an infectious agent through contaminated food, water, drugs, or blood

MATCHING 3-2: ACTIVITY EXAMPLE AND MEANS OF TRANSMISSION

Draw an arrow from the example of an activity that could lead to infection in column one to the most likely means of transmission that would be involved in column two. Use a different colored pen or pencil for each arrow. Answers can be used only once.

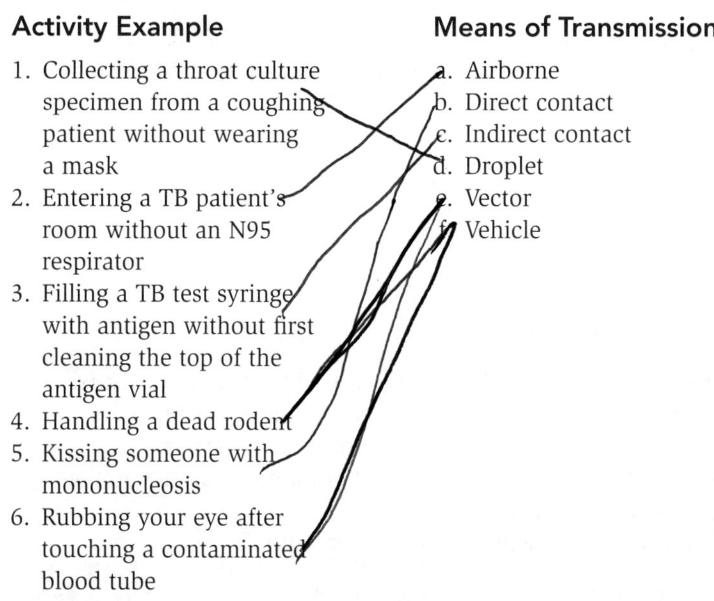

Activity Example	Means of Transmission
1. Collecting a throat culture specimen from a coughing patient without wearing a mask	a. Airborne
2. Entering a TB patient's room without an N95 respirator	b. Direct contact
3. Filling a TB test syringe with antigen without first cleaning the top of the antigen vial	c. Indirect contact
4. Handling a dead rodent	d. Droplet
5. Kissing someone with mononucleosis	e. Vector
6. Rubbing your eye after touching a contaminated blood tube	f. Vehicle

MATCHING 3-3: CLASS OF FIRE, TYPE OF MATERIAL, AND METHOD REQUIRED TO EXTINGUISH

Using a different colored pen or pencil for each class of fire, draw an arrow from the class of fire in the first column to the type of materials involved in the second column. Using the same color used for the class of fire, draw an arrow from the type of material involved to the method required to extinguish the fire found in the third column.

Class of Fire	Type of Material	Method Required to Extinguish
Class A	1. Combustible metals	a. Block oxygen source or smother
Class B	2. Electrical equipment	b. Cool and smother with splash prevention agent
Class C	3. Flammable liquid	c. Cool with water or water-based solution
Class D	4. Cooking oils	d. Extinguish with dry powder agent or sand
Class K	5. Wood or paper	e. Extinguish with nonconducting agent

MATCHING 3-4: TYPE OF SPILL AND CLEANUP PROCEDURE

Match the type of spill with the cleanup procedure (text Procedure 3-2).

Type of Spill

1. _____ small spill (a few drops)
2. _____ large spill
3. _____ dried spill
4. _____ spill involving broken glass

Cleanup Procedure

A. Carefully absorb spill with a paper towel or similar material. Discard material in biohazard waste container. Clean area with appropriate disinfectant.
B. Moisten spill with disinfectant (avoid scraping, which could disperse infectious organisms into the air). Absorb spill with paper towel or similar material. Discard material in biohazard waste container. Clean area with appropriate disinfectant.
C. Use a special clay or chlorine-based powder to absorb or gel (thicken) the liquid. Scoop or sweep up absorbed or thickened material. Discard material in a biohazard waste container. Wipe spill area with appropriate disinfectant.
D. Wear heavy-duty utility gloves. Scoop or sweep up material. Discard in biohazard sharps container. Clean area with appropriate disinfectant.

Labeling Exercises

LABELING EXERCISE 3-1: NFPA 704 MARKING SYSTEM

Label the quadrants in the NFPA marking system diagram below according to the type of hazard they identify. Color the quadrants the appropriate color code (one quadrant will remain uncolored). Using a black marker, write the signal number (or draw the symbol if applicable) for each of the following hazards in the appropriate quadrant:

- Material that on short exposure could cause serious temporary injury even with prompt medical attention
- Material that would have to be preheated before ignition could occur
- Material that is capable of detonating or exploding at normal temperature and pressure
- Material that is radioactive

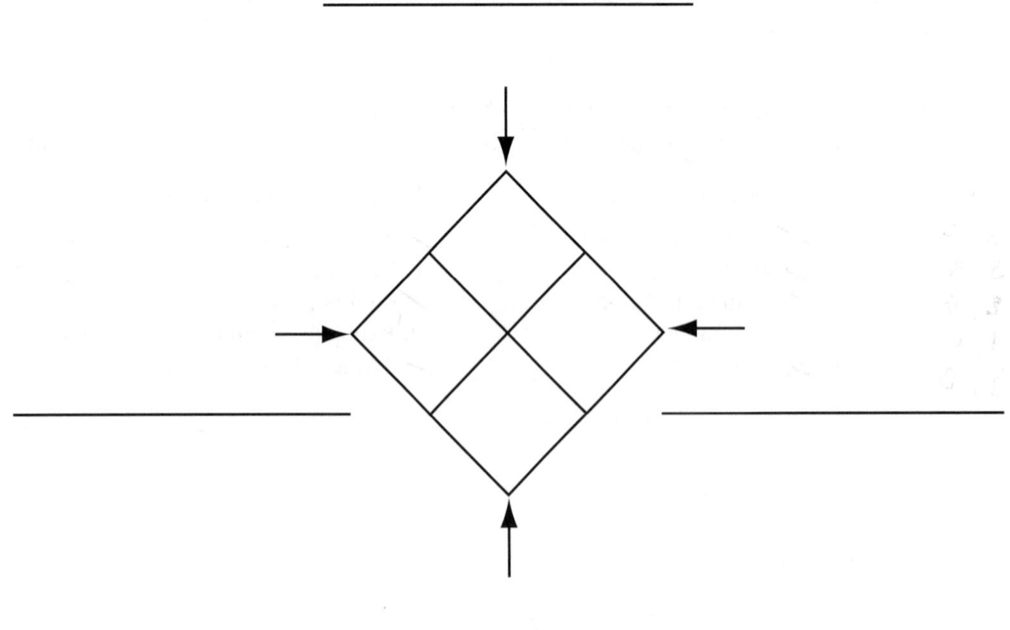

LABELING EXERCISE 3-2: ENGINEERING CONTROLS AND WORK PRACTICE CONTROLS

Each illustration below shows an engineering control, work practice control, or both. Write what the illustration shows and the control type(s) shown on the corresponding line beneath the illustration.

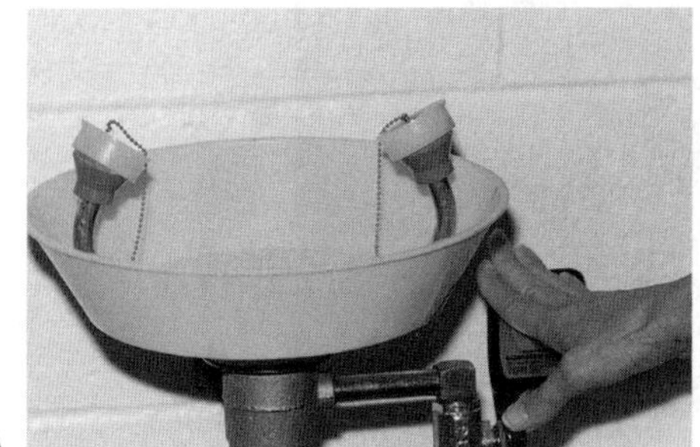
A

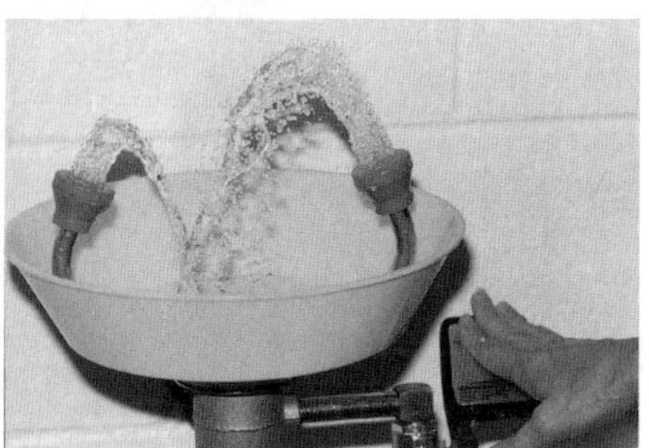
B

1. ______________________________

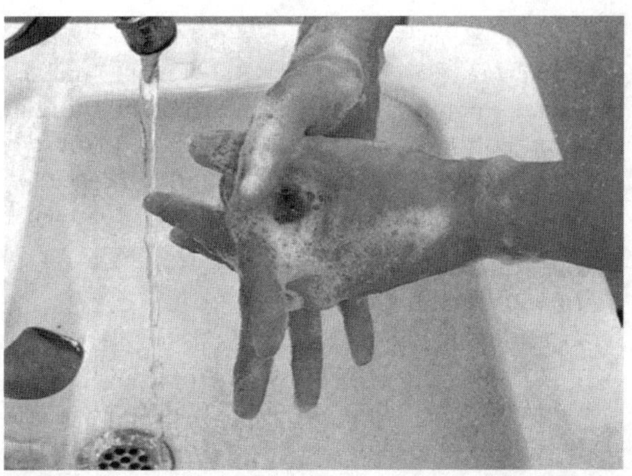

2. ______________________________

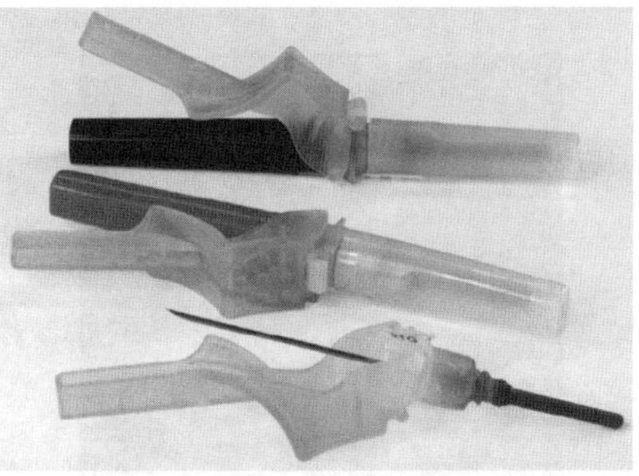

3. ______________________________

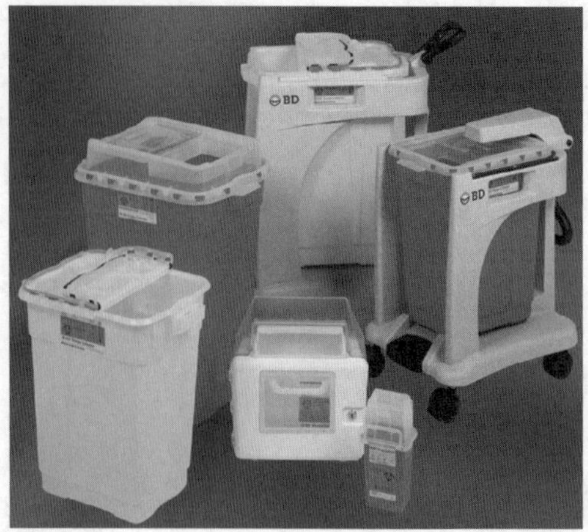

4. ______________________________

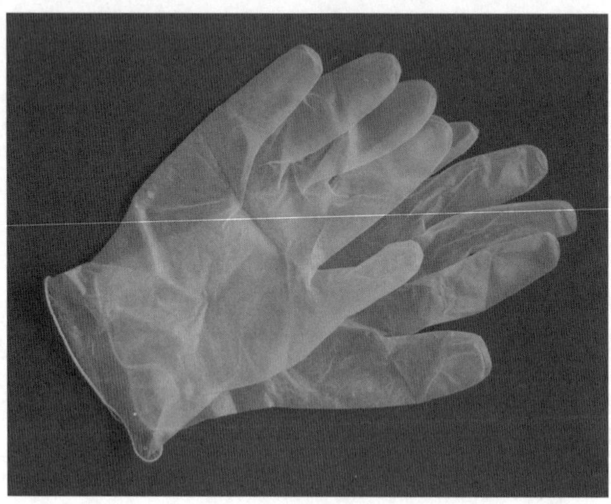

5. ______________________________

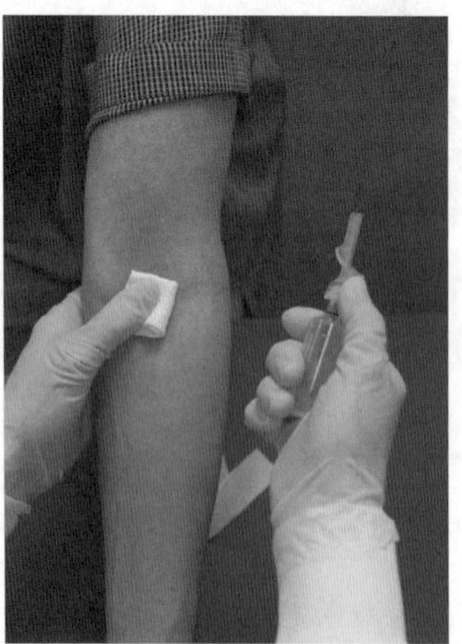

6. ______________________________

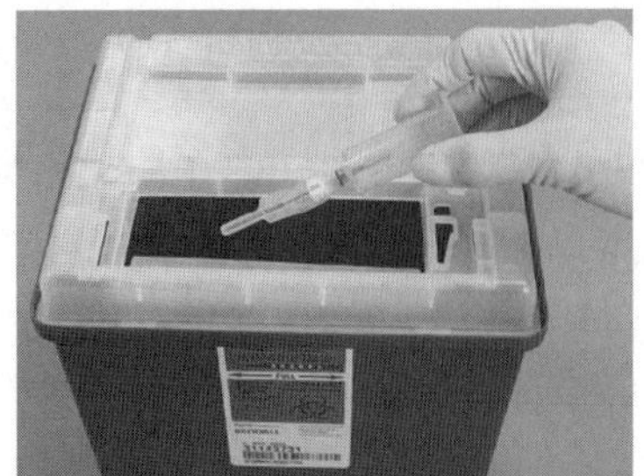

7. ______________________________

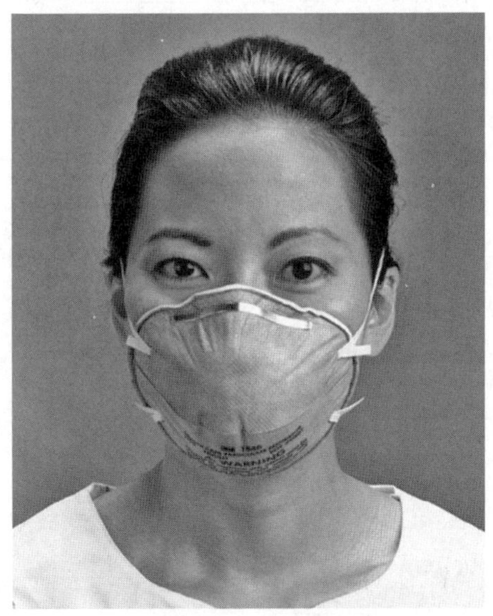

8. ______________________________

Knowledge Drills

KNOWLEDGE DRILL 3-1: CAUTION AND KEY POINT RECOGNITION

The following sentences are taken from selected Caution and Key Point statements found throughout the Chapter 3 text. Using the textbook, fill in the blanks with the missing information.

1. The transmission of (A) ____________ viruses and (B) ____________ through blood transfusion is also considered (C) ____________ transmission.
2. (A) ____________ transmission differs from airborne transmission in that (B) ____________ do not normally travel more than (C) ____________ and do not remain (D) ________________ in the air.
3. Individuals who are exposed to the (A) ________________________ are less likely to contract the disease if they have previously completed an (B) ___________________ series.
4. (A) ___________________ regulations require employers to offer (B) ______________________ free of charge to (C) __________________ whose duties involve risk of (D) __________________.
5. As part of the (A) ____________ *Guidelines for Hand Hygiene in Health Care Settings,* it is recommended that artificial (B) ____________ or (C) ___________________ not be worn when having direct contact with (D) ____________ patients, such as infants or those in ICU.
6. Wearing (A) ____________ during phlebotomy procedures is (B) ____________ by the OSHA (C) ____________ ____________ ____________.
7. The (A) ____________ standard is known as The Right to (B) ____________ law because of the (C) ____________ requirement.
8. The original compress should not be removed when adding (A) ____________ ones because removal can (B) ____________ the (C) ____________ process.
9. *Never* give fluids if the patient is (A) ___________________ or (B) ___________________ or has injuries likely to require (C) ____________ and anesthesia.
10. If activity during work is low to moderate AICR recommends that a person take an hour's (A) ____________ ____________ or similar exercise (B) ____________ because there has been convincing evidence that (C) ____________ ____________ helps prevent (D) ____________ cancer.
11. If hands are heavily contaminated with (A) ____________ material and hand-washing facilities are not available, it is recommended that hands be cleaned with (B) ____________ ____________ followed by the use of an (C) ___________________ antiseptic hand cleaner.
12. According to the CDC, (A) _________ _________ _________ is the most common (B) __________________ infection in the United States, accounting for (C) ____________ of all healthcare-associated infections.

KNOWLEDGE DRILL 3-2: SCRAMBLED WORDS

Use each numbered hint below to unscramble the words listed after it. Write the correct spelling of the scrambled word on the line next to it.

1. Three types of exposure routes
   a. merpuscola ______
   b. troucanesupe ______
   c. tegionnis ______
2. Together they create the need for a fire extinguisher
   a. teha ______
   b. genoxy ______
   c. lufe ______
   d. mechlica noriteac ______
3. They play a role in radiation exposure
   a. miet ______
   b. gleindish ______
   c. staindec ______
4. A chemical safety requirement
   a. ramtaile ______
   b. Yesfat ______
   c. taad ______
   d. hetse______
5. A symptom of shock
   a. pardi ______
   b. akew______
   c. slupe______
6. They play a role in personal wellness
   a. sciereex ______
   b. tunionirt ______
   c. neighey ______

KNOWLEDGE DRILL 3-3: BREAKING THE CHAIN OF INFECTION (Text Box 3-1)

List five things a phlebotomist can personally do to break the chain of infection.

1. ______________________
2. ______________________
3. ______________________
4. ______________________
5. ______________________

KNOWLEDGE DRILL 3-4: SITUATIONS THAT REQUIRE HAND HYGIENE

The following are statements concerning situations that require hand washing. Fill in the blanks with the missing information.

1. Before and after each ______________________
2. Between ______________________ procedures such as wound care and drawing blood
3. Before putting on gloves and ______________________
4. Before leaving the ______________________
5. Before going to lunch or ______________________
6. Before and after going to the ______________________
7. Whenever hands become ______________________ contaminated

KNOWLEDGE DRILL 3-5: SAFETY RULES WHEN IN PATIENT ROOMS AND OTHER PATIENT AREAS

The following are safety rules to follow when in patient rooms and other patient areas. After each rule, list at least one reason why it should be followed.

1. Avoid running. ______________________

   ____
2. Be careful entering and exiting patient rooms. ______________________
3. Do not touch electrical equipment in patient rooms while drawing blood. ______________________
4. Follow standard precautions when handling specimens. ______________________

   ____
5. Replace bed rails that were let down during patient procedures. ______________________

KNOWLEDGE DRILL 3-6: PATHOGEN TRANSMISSION AND PRECAUTIONS

A list of microorganisms follows. Using colored pens or pencils write "A" in blue next to airborne pathogens, and "B" in red next to bloodborne pathogens. Write "C" in black next to pathogens that require contact precautions, and "D" in green next to those that require droplet precautions

1. __C__ *C. difficile*
2. __B__ CMV
3. __C__ group A strep
4. __B__ HBV
5. __B__ HCV
6. __B__ HIV
7. __B__ HDV
8. __B__ malaria causing microbe
9. __B__ *Neisseria meningitidis*
10. __C__ RSV
11. __A__ rubeola virus
12. __C__ staph bacteria
13. __B__ syphilis-causing microbe
14. __A__ *Mycobacterium tuberculosis*
15. __A__ varicella virus

Skills Drills

SKILLS DRILL 3-1: REQUISITION ACTIVITY

A phlebotomist is sent to collect the specimens on the following requisition. Upon arrival at the patient's room, he finds an airborne precautions sign on the door.

Any Hospital USA
1123 West Physician Drive
Any Town USA

Laboratory Test Requisition

PATIENT INFORMATION:

Name: Doe (last) Jane (first) (MI)

Identification Number: 093656321 Birth Date: 04/11/68

Referring Physician: Payne

Date to be Collected: 03/15/11 Time to be Collected: 0600

Special Instructions: ______

TEST(S) REQUIRED:

____ NH4 – Ammonia	____ Gluc – glucose
____ Bili – Bilirubin, total & direct	____ Hgb – hemoglobin
____ BMP – basic metabolic panel	____ Lact – lactic acid/lactate
____ BUN – Blood urea nitrogen	____ Plt. Ct. – platelet count
____ Lytes – electrolytes	____ PT – prothrombin time
X CBC – complete blood count	____ PTT – partial thromboplastin time
____ Chol – cholesterol	____ RPR – rapid plasma reagin
X ESR – erythrocyte sed rate	____ T&S – type and screen
____ ETOH – alcohol	____ PSA – prostatic specific antigen
____ D-dimer	Other AFB culture

1. What precautions, if any, must the phlebotomist take before entering the room?
2. Which test requested might be a clue as to why the patient has airborne precautions?
3. What is the full name of the correct answer to #2 and why is it a clue to required precautions?
4. Name the disease the patient has, or is suspected of having?

SKILLS DRILL 3-2: WORD BUILDING

Divide each word below into all of its elements (parts): prefix (P), word root (WR), combining vowel (CV), and suffix (S). Write the word part, its definition, and the meaning of the word on the corresponding lines. If the word does not have a particular element, write NA (not applicable) in its place.

Example: neonatal

Elements ___*neo*___ / ___*nat*___ / ______ / ___*al*___
P WR CV S

Definitions ___*new*___ / ___*birth*___ / ______ / ___*pertaining to*___

Meaning: pertaining to a newborn

1. **Cardiopulmonary**

Elements ________ / ________ / ______ / ________ / ______
P WR CV WR S

Definition ________ / ________ / ______ / ________ / ______

Meaning:

2. **Dermatitis**

Elements ________ / ________ / ______ / ________ / ______
P WR CV S

Definition ________ / ________ / ______ / ________ / ______

Meaning:

3. **Hemorrhage**

Elements ________ / ________ / ______ / ________ / ______
P WR CV S

Definition ________ / ________ / ______ / ________ / ______

Meaning:

4. **Hepatitis**

Elements ________ / ________ / ______ / ________ / ______
P WR CV S

Definition ________ / ________ / ______ / ________ / ______

Meaning:

5. **Percutaneous**

Elements ________ / ________ / ______ / ________ / ______
P WR CV S

Definition ________ / ________ / ______ / ________ / ______

Meaning:

SKILLS DRILL 3-3: HAND-WASHING TECHNIQUE (Text Procedure 3-1)

Fill in the blanks with the missing information.

Step	Explanation/Rationale
1. Stand back so that you do not (A) ___________.	The (B) ___________ may be ___________ (C).
2. Turn on the faucet and (D) ___________ under warm, running water.	Water should not be too hot or (E)___________ and hands should be (F) ___________ before applying (G) ___________ to minimize drying, chapping, or cracking of hands from frequent hand washing.
3. Apply soap and work up a (H) ___________.	A good (I) ___________ is needed to reach all surfaces.
4. Scrub all surfaces, including between the fingers and around the (J) ___________.	Scrubbing is necessary to dislodge (K) ___________ from surfaces, especially between fingers and around (L) ___________.
5. Rub your hands together (M) ___________.	Friction helps loosen dead skin, dirt, debris, and (N) ___________. (Steps 4 and 5 should take at least (O) ___________, about the time it takes to sing the (P) ___________.)
6. Rinse your hands in a (Q)___________ motion from (R) ___________ to (S) ___________.	Rinsing with the hands (T) ___________ allows (U) ___________ to be (V) ___________ of the hands and fingers into the sink rather than flowing (W) ___________ the arm or wrist.
7. Dry hands with a (X) ___________ paper towel.	Hands must be dried thoroughly and gently to prevent chapping or cracking. (Y) ___________ towels can be a source of (Z)___________.
8. Use a (AA) ___________ paper towel to (BB) ___________ unless it is foot or motion activated.	Clean hands should not touch contaminated (CC)___________.

Crossword

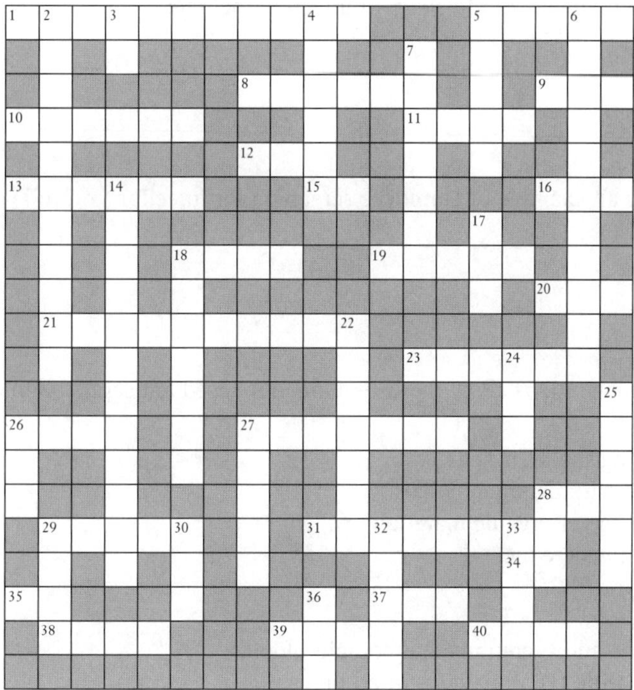

ACROSS

1. Condition showing decreased amount of neutrophils
5. Types of fire, ________ A, B, C, D or K
8. Bio________, security when handling biological materials
9. Incorporated disease- and category-specific precautions
10. Capable of living
11. Pathway link in the chain of infection
12. Federal agency charged with controlling disease
13. Infectious insect, arthropod, or animal
15. Tuberculosis
16. Tuberculin test
18. PPE facial covering
19. Results from insufficient blood flow to the heart
20. Most frequently occurring lab-related blood-borne pathogen
21. Infection acquired in the hospital
23. Resistant to a disease
26. Code used to remember how to operate a fire extinguisher
27. Preparation to prevent acquiring a disease
28. AIDS virus
29. Institute requiring N95 respirator for HCWs who may encounter airborne contaminants
31. __________ precautions
34. Intravenous (abbrev.)
35. CDC guidelines to prevent exposure to BBPs
37. Environmental protection agency (abbrev.)
38. Institute that suggests a predominantly plant-based diet
39. Protective covering for skin and clothing
40. Percutaneous means through the________.

DOWN

2. OSHA requires ____________devices
3. An N95 respirator must be worn around a patient with this disease
4. Cause to become diseased with virus or bacteria
5. __________ of infection
6. Having little resistance to infection or disease
7. Basin for flushing eye after contamination
14. Process of passing disease from one to another
17. Unit in a hospital where intensive care is given
18. Microscopic organism
22. An example of PPE clothing worn over scrubs
24. Most common nosocomial infection
25. PPEs for hands
26. Tuberculin test
27. Type of agent for hepatitis disease
28. Anyone infected with HBV is at risk for acquiring this virus
29. Agency that regulates fire codes
30. Most widespread chronic blood-borne illness in the United States
32. For example, microorganism capable of producing disease
33. Chance of injury, damage or loss
36. Federal agency dealing with transportation

Chapter Review Questions

1. Terms used to identify components of the chain of infection include:
   a. Infectious agent
   b. Susceptible host
   c. Reservoir
   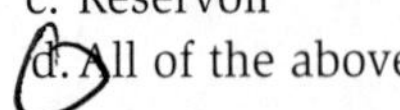
   d. All of the above

2. Which of the following is an example of employee screening for infection control?
   a. HBV vaccination
   b. MMR vaccination
   c. TB testing
   d. All of the above

3. CDC and HICPAC recommendations allow the use of alcohol-based antiseptic hand cleaners in place of hand washing as long as
   a. gloves were worn during the prior activity.
   b. hands are first cleaned with detergent wipes.
   c. hands have no visible dirt or organic material.
   d. all of the above conditions are met.

4. Standard precautions:
   a. apply only to secretions and excretions that contain blood.
   b. are to be used when caring for all patients at all times.
   c. never supersede other CDC isolation recommendations.
   d. should not be combined with other precautions.

5. Which of the following actions would violate a lab safety rule?
   a. Chewing gum while processing specimens
   b. Keeping food in a lab reagent refrigerator
   c. Wearing artificial nails
   d. All of the above

6. Which of the following is an example of a blood-borne pathogen?
   a. Cytomegalovirus
   b. Group A strep
   c. TB mycobacterium
   d. Varicella virus

7. Which of the following meet the OSHA BBP standard definition of an engineering control?
   a. Self-sheathing needle
   b. Sharps container
   c. Splash shield
   d. All of the above

8. The best defense against HBV infection is:
   a. HBV vaccination.
   b. proper hand hygiene.
   c. using safety needles.
   d. wearing gloves.

9. Which of the following involves the possibility of a permucosal BBP exposure?
   a. Failing to cover broken skin with a bandage
   b. Getting stuck with a used phlebotomy needle
   c. Licking the fingers to turn lab manual pages
   d. Opening blood tubes without a safety shield

10. Proper procedure for cleaning the site of an injury from a contaminated needle includes:
    a. cleaning it with povidone–iodine or other antiseptic.
    b. squeezing the injured area hard until it bleeds freely.
    c. washing it with soap and water for at least 30 seconds.
    d. all of the above.

11. Class "C" fires occur with:
    a. ordinary combustibles.
    b. flammable liquids.
    c. electrical equipment.
    d. reactive metals.

12. Normally the most effective means of controlling external hemorrhage is:
    a. application of a tourniquet.
    b. applying firm direct pressure.
    c. finger pressure over an artery.
    d. holding an ice pack on the site.

13. In the event of a chemical splash to the eyes, they should be flushed with water for:
    a. 2 minutes.
    b. 5 minutes.
    c. 10 minutes.
    d. 15 minutes.

14. In the NFPA 704 marking system, health hazards are indicated in the:
    a. blue quadrant on the left.
    b. red quadrant at the top.
    c. yellow quadrant on the right.
    d. white quadrant on the bottom.

15. Approximately 20% of all workplace injuries involve:
    a. back injuries.
    b. foot problems.
    c. needlesticks.
    d. stress reactions.

CASE STUDIES

Case Study 3-1 Airborne Precautions

A phlebotomist arrives at a patient's room for a timed blood draw. She observes an airborne precautions sign on the patient's door. There is a cart in the hallway outside the door with supplies on it.

QUESTIONS

1. What will the phlebotomist have to do before she enters the room? PUT ON REQUIRE PPE THATS APPROPRIATE FOR THE ROOM.
2. Will the specimen require special handling in addition to what is normally required for the test?
3. Name one disease that requires airborne precautions for anyone entering the patient's room.
4. Name two diseases that do not require airborne precautions for a phlebotomist who is immune to them.

Case Study 3-2 Work Restrictions (textbook Appendix D)

A phlebotomist wakes up with a fever and an extremely sore throat. He calls his physician who sends him to a lab for a rapid strep test. The test is positive for group A strep. The physician gives him a prescription for an antibiotic. The phlebotomist picks up the prescription and takes the first dose at 1300 hours. He is scheduled to work later that afternoon. He has used all his sick leave so he takes some aspirin and goes to work.

QUESTIONS

1. What work restrictions are required for a person with strep throat?
2. What is the earliest that he should have reported for work provided he was symptom free?
3. What might be the consequences of reporting to work when he still had symptoms?

(3-1)

①

② NO

③ TB

④ ~~TB, HBV~~ CHICKEN POX RUBELLA

(3-2)

① ~~AIRBORNE~~ / STAY HOME NO WORK

② 24 hrs FROM 1300 hrs

③ GETTING PT'S SICK.

UNIT I CROSSWORD EXERCISE

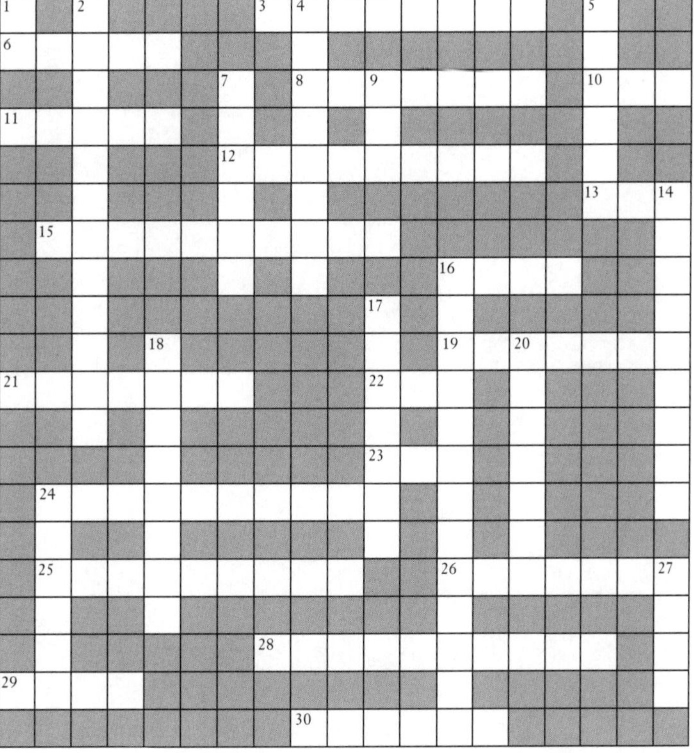

ACROSS

3. Type of disease transmission that disperses the infectious agent in evaporated droplet nuclei
6. *Exsanguinated* means that all of this is removed
8. Inanimate objects that harbor material containing infectious agent
10. Center for Medicare and Medicaid Services initials
11. Federal law that was designed to regulate patient privacy (abbrev.)
12. Preestablished value indicating a level of acceptable practice
13. College of American Pathologists initials
15. Compares current lab results on a patient with previous results for the same test
16. Global, nonprofit standards-developing organization
19. A neutropenic patient may be placed in this type of isolation
21. Level of care that should be exercised in the given circumstances
22. Hematocrit (abbrev.)
23. Fluid found in the spinal column and around the brain (abbrev.)
24. Term used to describe an infection acquired in a hospital
25. Source of an infectious microorganism
26. An act or threat that causes one to be in fear of immediate battery
28. A process in which a party in a legal action is questioned under oath
29. Required of manufacturers to furnish on each of their products
30. Protected from or resistant to a particular disease or infection

DOWN

1. Antibody (abbrev.)
2. Educational standards for programs such as phlebotomy
4. Type of consent for a medical procedure that is voluntary and competent
5. Hospital advisory committee for infection-control (abbrev.)
7. Percutaneous exposures occur through this type of skin
9. New title for Clinical Laboratory Scientist (CLS) (abbrev.)
14. The study of an individual's concept and use of space
16. Evidence that fundamental competencies in a particular field have been mastered
17. Means of transmission through food or water
18. Microbe capable of causing disease
20. Microbes responsible for certain diseases such as the common cold
24. Health professionals who give direct patient care
27. Wrongful act against one's person

UNIT II OVERVIEW OF THE HUMAN BODY

CHAPTER 4

Medical Terminology

OBJECTIVES

Study the information in your textbook that corresponds to each objective to prepare yourself for the activities in this chapter.

1. Define the key terms listed at the beginning of this chapter.
2. Identify basic word elements individually and within medical terms.
3. State the meanings of common word roots, prefixes, and suffixes and identify unique plural endings.
4. State the meanings of medical terms composed of elements found in this chapter.
5. Demonstrate proper pronunciation of medical terms by using the general pronunciation guidelines found in this chapter.
6. State the meanings of common medical abbreviations listed in this chapter.
7. Identify items currently on the Joint Commission "Do Not Use" List and the list of items for possible future inclusion on the "Do Not Use" List.

Matching

Use choices only once unless otherwise indicated.

MATCHING 4-1: KEY TERMS AND DESCRIPTIONS

Match each key term with the *best* description.

Key Terms

1. ______ combining form
2. ______ combining vowel
3. ______ prefix
4. ______ suffix
5. ______ word root

Descriptions

A. Comes before a word root and modifies its meaning
B. Establishes the basic meaning of a medical term
C. Follows a word root and adds to or changes the meaning
D. Identifies the plural form of a word
E. Makes pronunciation easier
F. Signifies a Latin word root
G. Word root joined with a vowel

MATCHING 4-2: WORD ROOTS AND MEANINGS

Match each word root with its meaning.

Word Roots

1. ______ chondr
2. ______ cry
3. ______ cyt
4. ______ glyc
5. ______ hemat
6. ______ lip
7. ______ my
8. ______ thromb
9. ______ ren
10. ______ scler

Meanings

A. Bladder
B. Blood
C. Bone
D. Cartilage
E. Cell
F. Chest
G. Clot
H. Cold
I. Fat
J. Hard
K. Kidney
L. Liver
M. Lung
N. Muscle
O. Pain
P. Sugar

MATCHING 4-3: PREFIXES AND MEANINGS

Match each prefix with its meaning.

Prefixes

1. ____ a-
2. ____ brady-
3. ____ epi-
4. ____ homeo-
5. ____ intra-
6. ____ macro-
7. ____ neo-
8. ____ per-
9. ____ poly-
10. ____ tri-

Meanings

A. Before
B. Between
C. Difficult
D. Equal
E. Large
F. Many
G. New
H. Outside
I. Over
J. Same
K. Slow
L. Three
M. Through
N. Unequal
O. Within
P. Without

MATCHING 4-4: SUFFIXES AND MEANINGS

Match each suffix with its meaning.

Suffixes

1. ____ -algia
2. ____ -emia
3. ____ -ic
4. ____ -ism
5. ____ -itis
6. ____ -lysis
7. ____ -meter
8. ____ -penia
9. ____ -stasis
10. ____ -tomy

Meanings

A. Blood condition
B. Breakdown
C. Bursting forth
D. Condition
E. Deficiency
F. Incision
G. Infection
H. Inflammation
I. Measuring instrument
J. Pain
K. Pertaining to
L. Recording
M. Specialist
N. Stopping
O. Tumor
P. Twitch

Labeling Exercises

LABELING EXERCISE 4-1: WORD ELEMENTS AND MEANINGS

Identify the highlighted element in each medical term listed below. Write the type of element (prefix, word root, combining vowel or form, or suffix) and its meaning on the corresponding line. If the element has no meaning, write NA.

Medical Term	Type of Element	Element Meaning
1. arteriospasm	SUFFIX	TWITCH
2. cyanotic	PRE	BLUE
3. cytology	VOWEL	
4. diapedesis	PREFIX	ACROSS
5. endocrinologist	WORD ROOT	TO SECRETE
6. hemopoiesis	SUFFIX	
7. neonatal	PREFIX	NEW
8. osteochrondritis	VOWEL	CARTILAGE
9. postprandial	COMBINING VOWEL	MEAL
10. tachycardia	PREFIX	RAPID

LABELING EXERCISE 4-2: SINGULAR AND PLURAL WORD ENDINGS

Highlight the word endings in each of the medical terms below and circle any that are plural. Write the applicable singular or plural form of the term on the corresponding line.

1. lumina LUMEN
2. ova OVUM
3. papillae PAPILLA
4. phalanx PHALANGES
5. protozoa PROTOZUM.

Knowledge Drills

KNOWLEDGE DRILL 4-1: KEY POINT RECOGNITION

The following sentences are taken from Key Point statements found in Chapter 4 of the textbook. Fill in the blanks with the missing information.

1. A (A) ________________ ________________ typically indicates a (B) ________________, organ, body system, color, condition, substance, or (C) ________________.
2. However, a combining (A) ________________ is kept between two (B) ________ ________, even if the second (C) ________________ begins with a vowel.
3. When a suffix begins with (A)________________, the (B) ________________ is (C) ________________ as in hemorrhage.
4. When a suffix is added to a word ending in (A) ________________, the (B) ________________ is changed to a (C) ________________, as in pharynx becoming (D) ________________ and (E) ________________ becoming thoracic.
5. It is more important to be able to identify the (A) __________ of a word (B) ________________ than to identify its (C) ________________.
6. To determine the meaning of a medical term, it is generally best to start with the (A) ________________, then go to the (B) ________________, and identify the meaning of the (C) ________________ or (D) ________________ last.
7. A (A) ________________ (B) ________________ is not normally used when a suffix starts with a (C) ________________.

KNOWLEDGE DRILL 4-2: SCRAMBLED WORDS

Unscramble the following words using the hints given in parenthesis. Write the correct spelling of the scrambled word on the line next to it.

1. thagolpoy ________________________ (the study of disease)
2. sloycligys ________________________ (breakdown of sugar)
3. pasedio ________________________ (pertaining to fat)
4. tucubansouse ________________________ (beneath the skin)
5. yendasp ________________________ (difficult breathing)
6. nelra ________________________ (pertaining to the kidneys)
7. vexalcasutrar ________________________ (outside the blood vessels)
8. cetryocmi ________________________ (a small cell)
9. trienesti ________________________ (intestinal inflammation)
10. critocles ________________________ (pertaining to being hard)

Skills Drills

SKILLS DRILL 4-1: REQUISITION ACTIVITY

The following requisition contains abbreviations for common laboratory tests. Write the full name of the test in the space provided on the requisition.

Any Hospital USA
1123 West Physician Drive
Any Town USA

Laboratory Test Requisition

PATIENT INFORMATION:

Name: ____________ (last) ____________ (first) ____________ (MI)

Identification Number: ____________ Birth Date: ____________

Referring Physician: ____________

Date to be Collected: ____________ Time to be Collected: ____________

Special Instructions: ____________

TEST(S) REQUIRED:

Test	Full name	Test	Full name
ASO	ANTISTREPTOLYSIN O	Hgb	HEMOGLOBIN
Bili	BILRUBIN	Lytes	ELECTROLYTES
CBC	COMPLETE BLOOD COUNT	O&P	OVA + PARACITE
Chol	CHOLESTOROL	PT	PROTHROMBIN TIME
CK	CREATINE KINASE	PTT	PARTIAL THROMBOPLASTINE TIME
DIC	DISSAMINATED INTRAVASCULAR COA	RBC	RED BLOOD COUNT
ESR	ERYTHROCYTE SEDIMINTATION RATE	RPR	RAPID PLASMA REAGIN
FSH	FOLLICLE STIMULATING HORMONE	TIBC	TOTAL IRON BINDING CAPACITY
Gluc	GLUCOSE	TSH	THRYROID STIMULATING HORMONE
GTT	GLUCOSE TOLERENCE TEST	UA	URINARY ANALYSIS

SKILLS DRILL 4-2: WORD BUILDING

Build medical terms for each definition listed below. Identify each word element, prefix (P), word root (WR), combining vowel (CV), or suffix (S) needed to build the term and write the meaning of each element on the appropriate line.

1. blood tumor HEMAT (WR) / OMA (S)
2. cutting the vein PHLEB (WR) / O (CV) / TOMY (S)
3. low blood sugar HYPO (P) / GLY (WR) / CEMIA (S)
4. condition of death NECR (WR) / OSIS (S)
5. inflammation of the liver HEPAT (WR) / ITIS (S)
6. clotting cell THROMB (WR) / O (CV) / CITE (S)
7. specialist in the study of disease PATH (WR) / O (CV) / LOGIST (S)
8. large cell MACRO (P) / CITE (S)
9. stopping blood (or blood flow) HEMAT (WR) / O (CV) / STABAGE (S)
10. pertaining to poison TOX (WR) / IC (S)

Crossword

ACROSS

1. Prefix meaning different
3. Word root meaning glucose
5. Fasting blood sugar (abbrev.)
6. Prefix meaning small
9. Prefix meaning difficult
10. Before surgery (abbrev.)
11. Prefix meaning half
12. Word root meaning heart
15. Word root meaning vein
16. Prefix meaning below
17. Word root meaning intestines
18. Word root meaning clot
21. Word root meaning disease
22. Word root meaning kidney
23. Word root meaning head
27. Glucose tolerance test (abbrev.)
28. Word root meaning bone
30. Word root meaning tumor
31. Suffix meaning abnormal flow
33. Prefix meaning around
34. Word root meaning brain
37. Word root meaning chest
40. Word root meaning fiber
42. Prefix meaning within
43. Suffix meaning tumor
45. Prefix meaning after
46. Suffix meaning enzyme

DOWN

1. Prefix meaning same
2. Erythrocyte sedimentation rate (abbrev.)
3. Word root meaning stomach
4. Prefix meaning through
5. Fever of unknown origin (abbrev).
7. Prefix meaning blue
8. Suffix meaning condition
9. Disseminated intravascular coagulation (abbrev.)
10. Word root meaning vein
13. Word root meaning joint
14. Word root meaning artery
19. Word root meaning kidney
20. Word root meaning liver
21. Word root meaning lung
24. Word root meaning air
25. Suffix meaning specialist in study of
26. Word root meaning vessel
27. Word root meaning sugar
29. Word root meaning hard
32. Word root meaning blood
35. Word root meaning death
36. Prefix meaning against
38. Word root meaning bile
39. Suffix meaning inflammation
41. Prefix meaning new
44. Prefix meaning poor

Chapter Review Questions

1. This word element establishes the basic meaning of a medical term.
   a. Combining form
   b. Prefix
   c. Suffix
   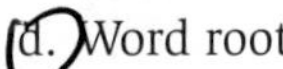
   d. Word root

2. Of the following word parts, which is a prefix?
   a. epi
   b. gram
   c. lip
   d. ole

3. To what part of the body does the word cephal refer?
   a. Kidney
   b. Head
   c. Intestine
   d. Liver

4. Which part of the word pericarditis is the word root?
   a. ardi
   b. cardi
   c. itis
   d. peri

5. What does the suffix *-lysis* mean?
   a. Breakdown
   b. Incision
   c. Stoppage
   d. Surgical puncture

6. The plural form of ovum is:
   a. ova.
   b. ovae.
   c. ovi
   d. ovix.

7. The singular form of atria is:
   a. atra.
   b. atrius.
   c. atrix.
   d. atrium.

8. The medical term for platelet is:
   a. coagulocyte.
   b. hepatocyte.
   c. leukocyte.
   d. thrombocyte.

9. Venule means:
   a. condition of a vein.
   b. pertaining to a vein.
   c. small vein.
   d. vein tumor.

10. Which of the following means kidney inflammation?
    a. Nephremia
    b. Nephritis
    c. Renemia
    d. Renitis

11. The "e" at the end is pronounced separately in:
    a. arteriole.
    b. flange.
    c. syncope.
    d. venule.

12. The abbreviation ESR stands for:
    a. erythrocyte sedimentation rate.
    b. established secondary reaction.
    c. estimated sedimentation range.
    d. evaluated survival response.

13. The abbreviation RBC means:
    a. random blood count.
    b. rare blood cancer.
    c. red blood cell.
    d. reduced blood content.

14. The abbreviation PPD means:
    a. platelet plasma donor.
    b. postprandial diet.
    c. potassium and phosphorus determination.
    d. purified protein derivative.

15. Which of the following abbreviations is on the Joint Commission's current "Do Not Use" List?
    a. ACTH
    b. HbSAg
    c. MSO_4
    d. PCO_2

CASE STUDIES

Case Study 4-1 Laboratory Orders

A phlebotomist receives a telephone order from the ICU requesting stat collection of ABGs, lytes, and a WBC on a patient with COPD.

QUESTIONS

1. What is the complete name of the patient's location?
2. What is the collection priority and what does it mean?
3. What are the complete names of the tests that the phlebotomist will collect?
4. What is the complete name of the disorder the patient has?

Case Study 4-2 Outpatient Blood Draw

A patient arrives at an outpatient surgery blood drawing station with a requisition from her physician for a pre-op CBC and a chem profile. The requisition indicates that the patient has h/o syncope and must be fasting for the tests and NPO for surgery, which is scheduled for later that morning.

QUESTIONS

1. Why is the patient having the blood tests?
2. What does NPO mean and how does the phlebotomist determine that the patient is NPO?
3. Look up the meaning of syncope in the glossary in the textbook. What does h/o syncope mean? Should it concern the phlebotomist? Why or why not?

(4-1)

① INTENSIVE CARE UNIT

② ABG's, LYTES, WBC, IMMEDIATELY

ARTERIAL BLOODGASES, WHITE BLOOD CELLS + COUNT, ELECTROLYTES

③ →

④ CHRONIC OBSTRUCTIVE PULMONARY DISEASE

(4-2)

① BECAUSES THERE GOING TO HAVE SURGERY (PRE-OP)

② NOTHING BY MOUTH, BY LOOKING AT THE RESTRICTIONS AND SEE SHE SHOULD BE FASTING, AND BY ASKING.

③ THE PAITENT HAS A HISTORY OF FAINTING, YES BECAUSE THEY DON'T WANT HE PASSING OUT.

CHAPTER

5

Human Anatomy and Physiology Review

OBJECTIVES

Study the information in your textbook associated with each objective to prepare yourself for the activities in this chapter.

1. Define the key terms and abbreviations listed at the beginning of this chapter.
2. Identify and describe body positions, planes, cavities, and directional terms.
3. Define homeostasis and the primary processes of metabolism.
4. Identify and describe the structural components of cells and the four basic types of body tissue.
5. Describe the function and identify the components or major structures of each body system.
6. List disorders and diagnostic tests commonly associated with each body system.

Matching

Use choices only once unless otherwise indicated.

MATCHING 5-1: KEY TERMS AND DESCRIPTIONS

Match each key term with the *best* description.

Key Terms (1–20)

1. ____ acidosis
2. ____ alkalosis
3. ____ alveoli
4. ____ anabolism
5. ____ anatomical position
6. ____ anatomy
7. ____ anterior
8. ____ avascular
9. ____ axons
10. ____ body cavities
11. ____ body plane
12. ____ bursae
13. ____ cartilage
14. ____ catabolism
15. ____ diaphragm
16. ____ distal
17. ____ dorsal
18. ____ endocrine glands
19. ____ exocrine glands
20. ____ frontal plane

Descriptions (1–20)

A. Air sacs in the lungs where exchange of gases takes place
B. Breakdown of complex substances into simple ones
C. Condition that results from a decrease in the pH of body fluids
D. Condition that results from an increase in the pH of body fluids
E. Conversion of simple compounds into complex substances
F. Farthest from the point of attachment
G. Flat surface of a real or imaginary cut through the body
H. Glands that secrete substances directly into the bloodstream
I. Glands that secrete substances through ducts
J. Hollow body spaces that house body organs
K. Means “at the back of the body or body part”
L. Muscle that separates the thoracic and abdominal cavities
M. Nerve fibers that conduct impulses away from the nerve cell body
N. Real or imaginary cut that divides the body vertically into front and back portions
O. Referring to the front
P. Small synovial fluid–filled sacs found near joints
Q. Standing erect with arms at the side and eyes and palms facing forward
R. Study of the structural composition of living things
S. Type of hard, nonvascular connective tissue
T. Without blood or lymph vessels

Key Terms (21–40)

21. ____ gametes
22. ____ hemopoiesis
23. ____ homeostasis
24. ____ hormones
25. ____ meninges
26. ____ metabolism
27. ____ mitosis
28. ____ nephron
29. ____ neuron
30. ____ phalanges

Descriptions (21–40)

A. Balanced or steady state
B. Chemical substances that affect many body processes
C. Connective tissue that encloses the brain and spinal chord
D. Divides the body horizontally into upper and lower portions
E. Divides the body vertically into right and left portions
F. Finger bones
G. Functional unit of the kidney
H. Fundamental unit of the nervous system
I. Gland secreting hormones that control other glands
J. Hollow spaces in the front of the body
K. Joint fluid
L. Lying face down and the act of turning face down
M. Lying face up and the act of turning face up
N. Nearest to the point of attachment
O. Process by which cells divide

31. __R__ physiology
32. __I__ pituitary gland
33. __L__ prone/pronation
34. __N__ proximal
35. __E__ sagittal plane
36. __M__ supine/supination
37. __S__ surfactant
38. __K__ synovial fluid
39. __D__ transverse plane
40. __J__ ventral cavities

P. Production of blood cells
Q. Sex cells
R. Study of the function of living things
S. Substance that coats the alveoli
T. Sum of all physical and chemical reactions that sustain life

MATCHING 5-2: STRUCTURES, DISORDERS, DIAGNOSTIC TESTS, AND BODY SYSTEMS

Match the structures, disorders, and diagnostic tests with the appropriate body systems. Choices may be used more than once.

Structures

1. __C__ biceps
2. __G__ bronchus
3. __H__ calcaneus
4. __D__ dendrite
5. __A__ esophagus
6. __F__ fallopian tube
7. __I__ glomerulus
8. __E__ papilla
9. __E__ sebaceous gland
10. __B__ thymus

Disorders

1. __C__ atrophy
2. __H__ bursitis
3. __E__ dermatitis
4. __B__ diabetes mellitus
5. __G__ emphysema
6. __A__ hepatitis
7. __B__ hypothyroidism
8. __D__ meningitis
9. __I__ nephritis
10. __F__ prostate cancer

Diagnostic Tests

1. __G__ AFB culture
2. __A__ bilirubin
3. __D__ CSF analysis
4. __C__ creatine kinase
5. __I__ creatinine clearance
6. __E__ skin scraping KOH prep
7. __A__ O&P
8. __F__ RPR
9. __B__ TSH
10. __H__ uric acid

Body Systems

A. Digestive
B. Endocrine
C. Muscular
D. Nervous
E. Integumentary
F. Reproductive
G. Respiratory
H. Skeletal
I. Urinary

Labeling Exercises

LABELING EXERCISE 5-1: BODY PLANES (Fig. 5-1)

Write the names of the three planes of division on the correct numbered lines in different colors. Then color each plane in the illustration with its corresponding color.

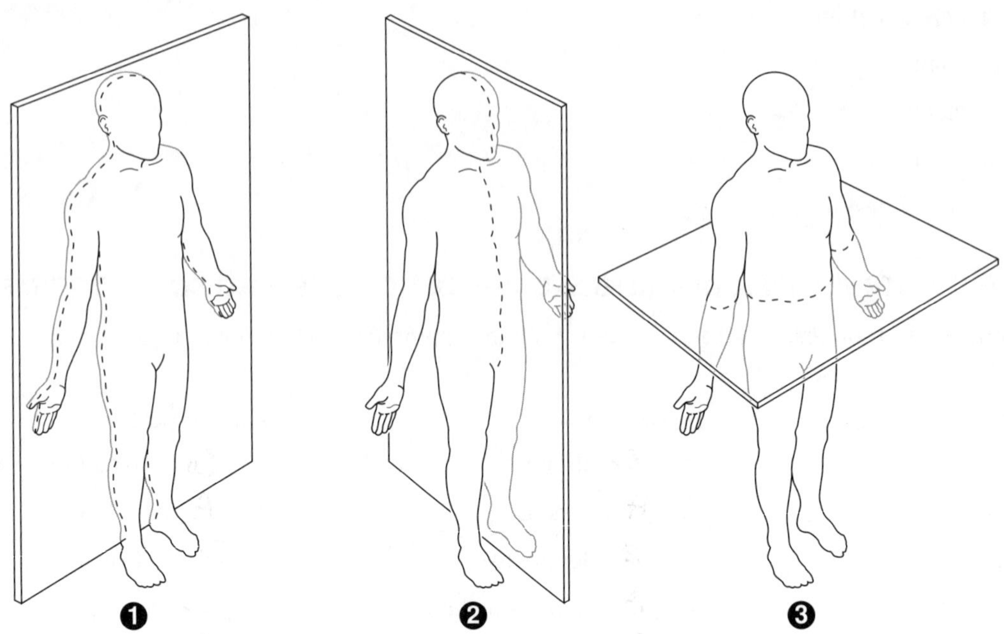

(Adapted with permission from BJ Cohen, KL Hull. *Study Guide for Memmler's the Human Body in Health and Disease,* 11th ed. Philadelphia: Lippincott Williams & Wilkins; 2009:7.)

1. ______________________________

2. ______________________________

3. ______________________________

LABELING EXERCISE 5-2: DIRECTIONAL TERMS (text Fig. 5-2)

Write the name of each directional term on the numbered lines in different colors. Then color the arrow corresponding to each directional term with the appropriate color.

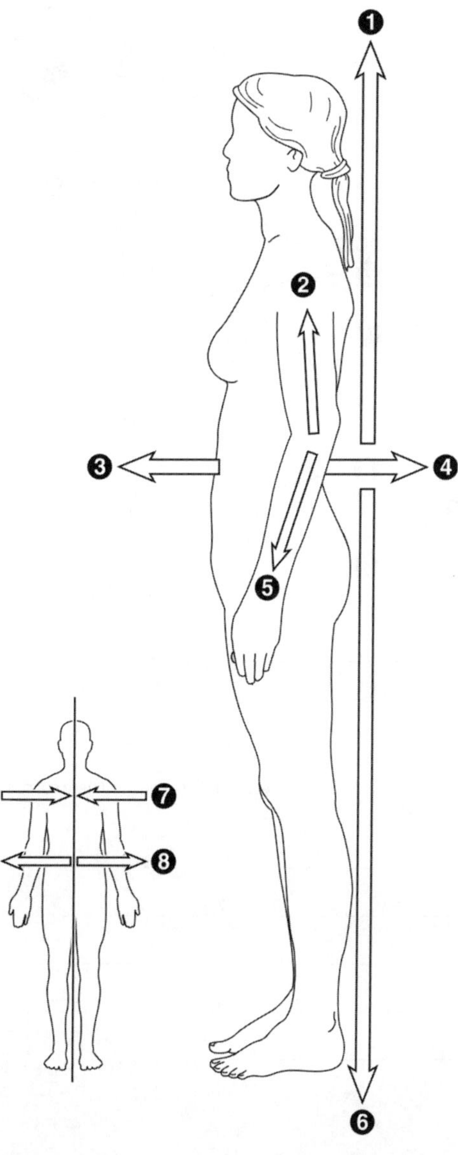

(Adapted with permission from BJ Cohen, KL Hull. *Study Guide for Memmler's the Human Body in Health and Disease,* 11th ed. Philadelphia: Lippincott Williams & Wilkins: 2009:6.)

1. ______________________
2. ______________________
3. ______________________
4. ______________________
5. ______________________
6. ______________________
7. ______________________
8. ______________________

LABELING EXERCISE 5-3: LATERAL VIEW OF BODY CAVITIES (text Fig. 5-3)

Identify the numbered body cavities and other structures and write the names on the corresponding lines below using different colors for each one. Then, color each cavity or structure with the color used to write the name.

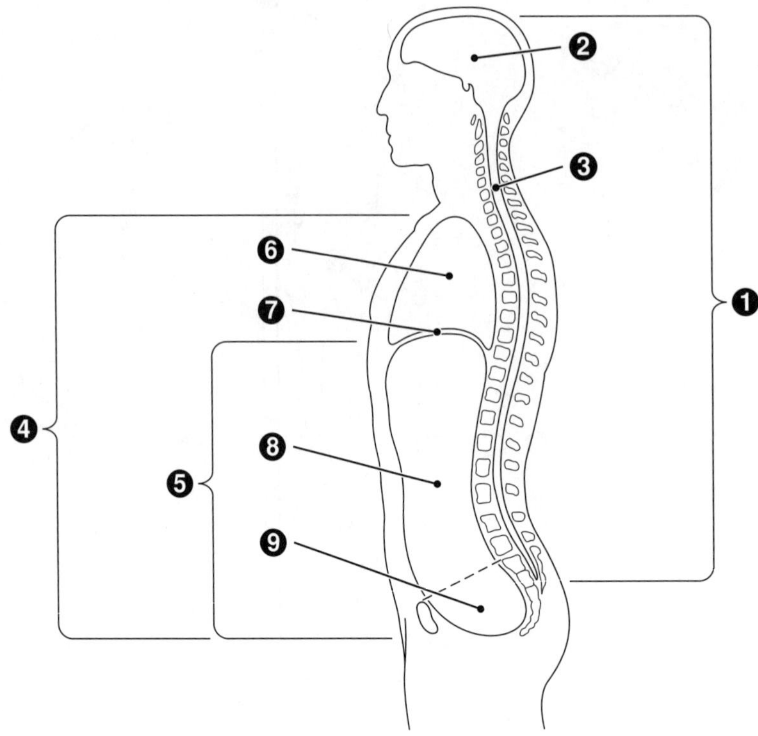

(Adapted with permission from BJ Cohen, KL Hull. *Study Guide for Memmler's the Human Body in Health and Disease,* 11th ed. Philadelphia: Lippincott Williams & Wilkins: 2009:8.)

1. ______________________
2. ______________________
3. ______________________
4. ______________________
5. ______________________
6. ______________________
7. ______________________
8. ______________________
9. ______________________

LABELING EXERCISE 5-4: CELL DIAGRAM (text Fig. 5-4)

Write the names of the numbered structures in different colors on the corresponding lines. Then color each structure with the color used to write the name.

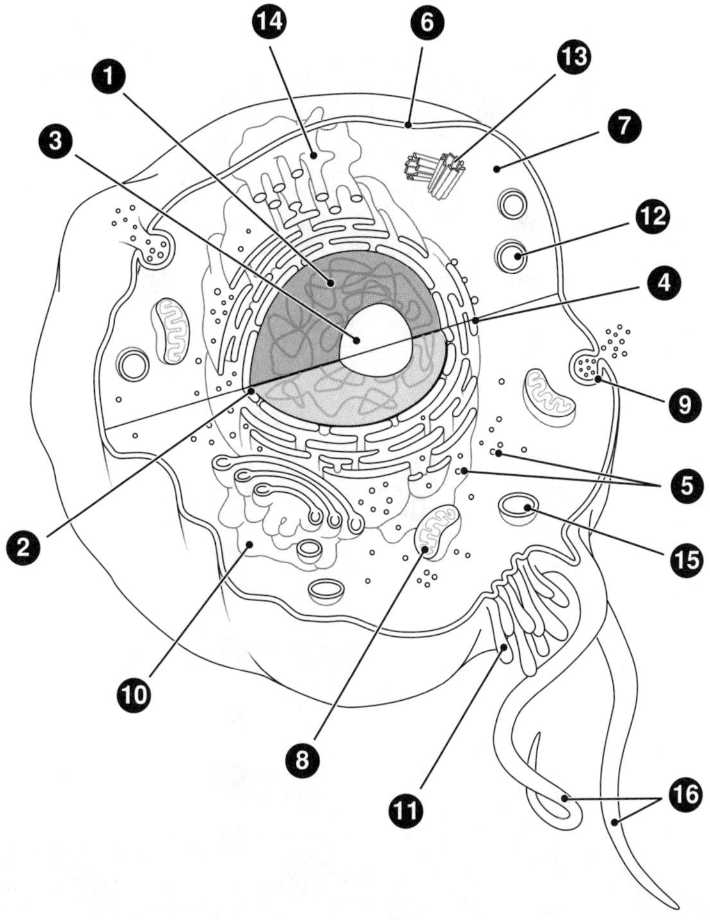

(Adapted with permission from BJ Cohen, KL Hull. *Study Guide for Memmler's the Human Body in Health and Disease,* 11th ed. Philadelphia: Lippincott Williams & Wilkins; 2009:38.)

1. ______________________
2. ______________________
3. ______________________
4. ______________________
5. ______________________
6. ______________________
7. ______________________
8. ______________________
9. ______________________
10. ______________________
11. ______________________
12. ______________________
13. ______________________
14. ______________________
15. ______________________
16. ______________________

LABELING EXERCISE 5-5: HUMAN SKELETON (text Fig. 5-5)

Write the name of each labeled part on the numbered lines in different colors. Use the same color for structures 19 and 20 and structures 24 and 25. Then color the different structures on the diagram with the corresponding color. Try to color every structure in the figure with the appropriate color. For instance, structure number 3 is found in two locations.

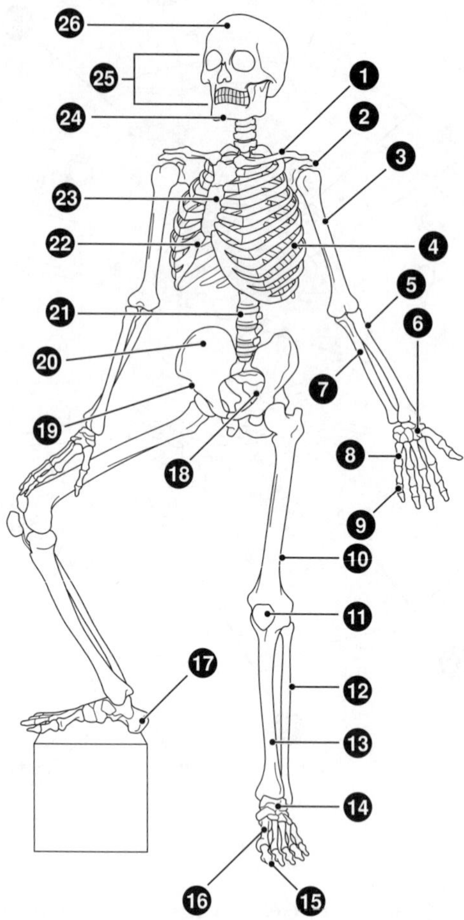

(Adapted with permission from BJ Cohen, KL Hull. *Study Guide for Memmler's the Human Body in Health and Disease,* 11th ed. Philadelphia: Lippincott Williams & Wilkins; 2009:111.)

1. ______________________
2. ______________________
3. ______________________
4. ______________________
5. ______________________
6. ______________________
7. ______________________
8. ______________________
9. ______________________
10. ______________________
11. ______________________
12. ______________________
13. ______________________
14. ______________________
15. ______________________
16. ______________________
17. ______________________
18. ______________________
19. ______________________
20. ______________________
21. ______________________
22. ______________________
23. ______________________
24. ______________________
25. ______________________
26. ______________________

LABELING EXERCISE 5-6: MUSCULAR SYSTEM (text Fig. 5-6)

Write the names of the three types of muscle tissue in the appropriate blanks using different colors. Color the muscle cells the corresponding color. Color the nuclei a different color. Draw arrows from the muscle picture to the corresponding site on the body.

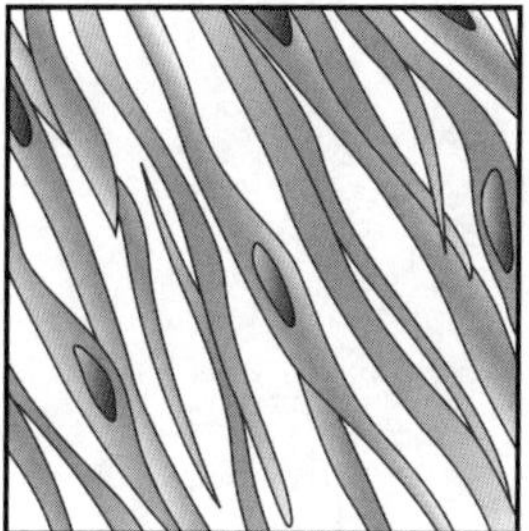

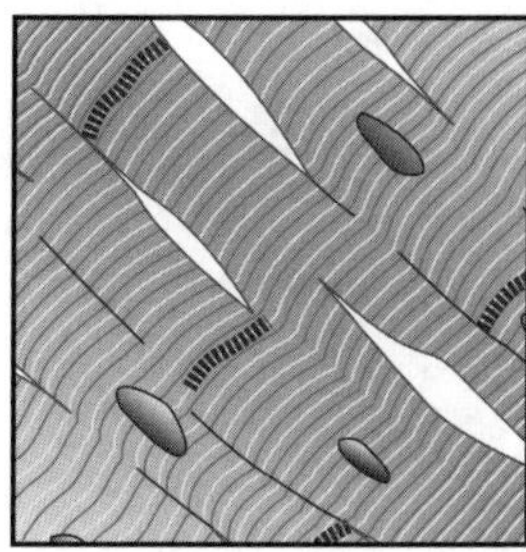

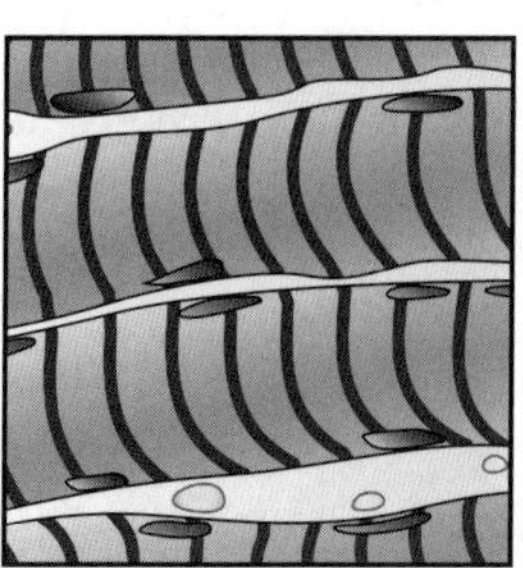

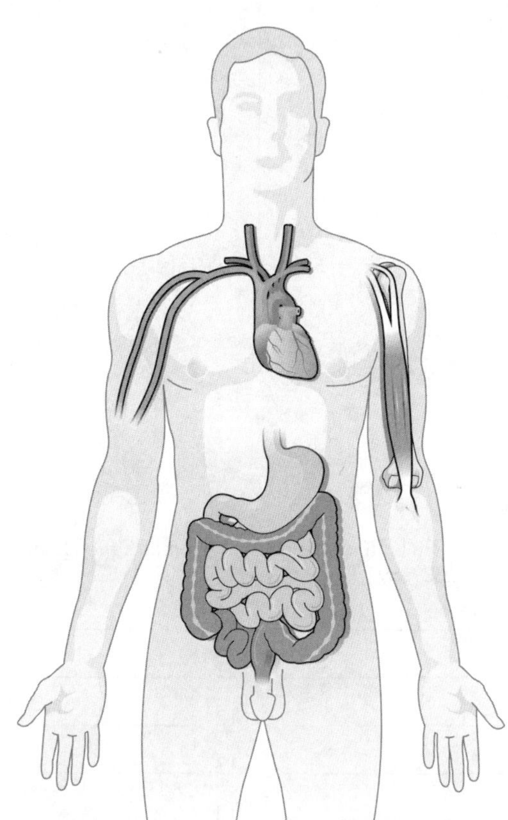

(Adapted with permission from BJ Cohen, KL Hull. *Study Guide for Memmler's the Human Body in Health and Disease,* 11th ed. Philadelphia: Lippincott Williams & Wilkins; 2009:54.)

1. ______________________________

2. ______________________________

3. ______________________________

LABELING EXERCISE 5-7: INTEGUMENTARY SYSTEM (text Fig. 5-7)

Identify the skin layers shown in numbers 1 through 3 and write the names in the corresponding boxes. Use different colors to write the names of the other numbered structures on the corresponding lines below. Use red if the structure is an artery and blue if it is a vein. Color the various structures within the diagram with the color used to write the name. Remember, some structures are found in more than one place.

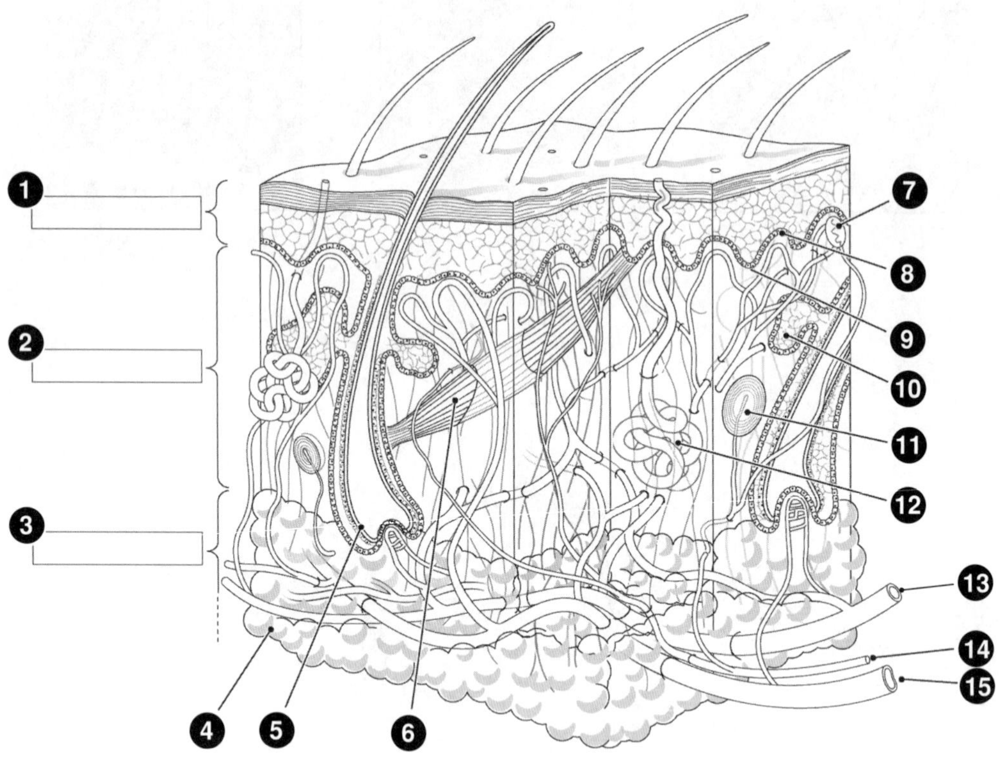

(Adapted with permission from BJ Cohen, KL Hull. *Study Guide for Memmler's the Human Body in Health and Disease,* 11th ed. Philadelphia: Lippincott Williams & Wilkins; 2009: 89.)

4. ______________________
5. ______________________
6. ______________________
7. ______________________
8. ______________________
9. ______________________
10. ______________________
11. ______________________
12. ______________________
13. ______________________
14. ______________________
15. ______________________

LABELING EXERCISE 5-8: NERVOUS SYSTEM (text Fig. 5-8)

Identify the numbered parts and divisions of the nervous system and write the names on the corresponding lines below.

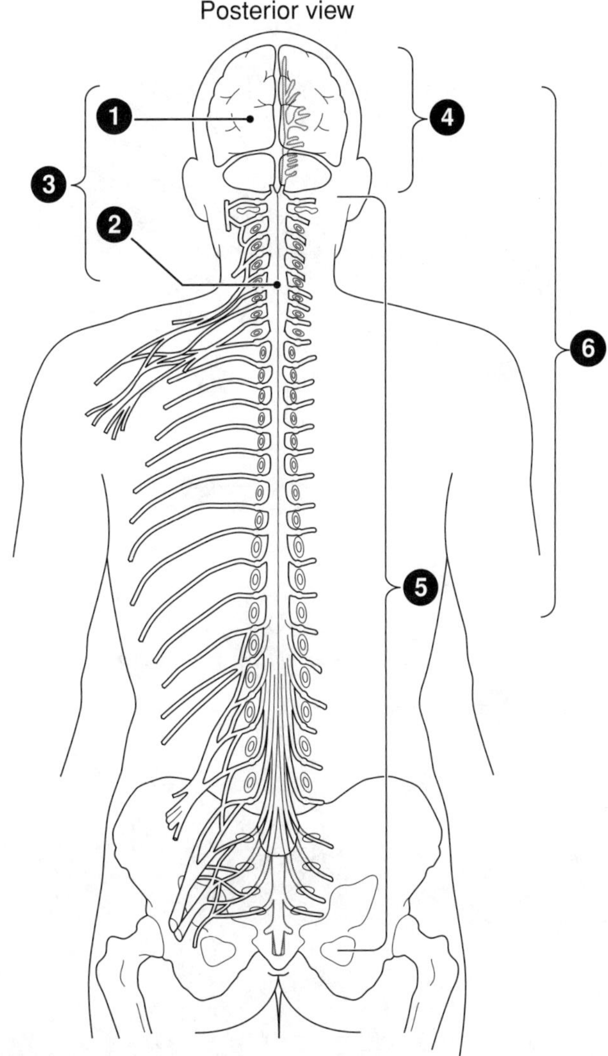

(Adapted with permission from BJ Cohen, KL Hull. *Study Guide for Memmler's the Human Body in Health and Disease,* 11th ed. Philadelphia: Lippincott Williams & Wilkins; 2009:149.)

1. ____________________
2. ____________________
3. ____________________
4. ____________________
5. ____________________
6. ____________________

LABELING EXERCISE 5-9: MOTOR NEURON (text Fig. 5-9)

Use different colors to write the names of the numbered structures on the corresponding lines below. Color the structures within the diagram the same colors used to write their names. Do not color structures 5 and 6. Add large arrows to the diagram showing the direction the nerve impulse will travel to get from the dendrites to the muscle.

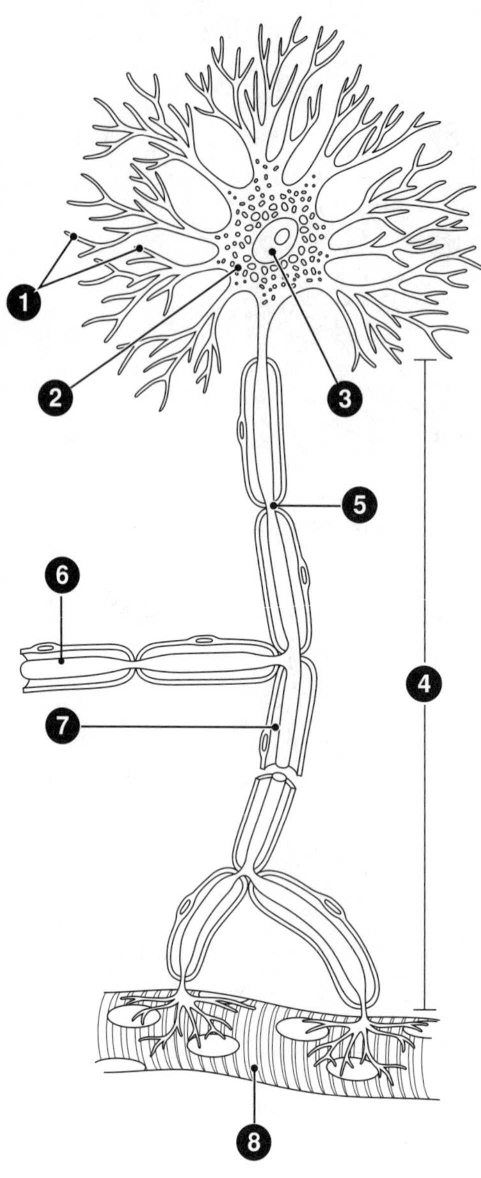

(Adapted with permission from BJ Cohen, KL Hull. *Study Guide for Memmler's the Human Body in Health and Disease,* 11th ed. Philadelphia: Lippincott Williams & Wilkins; 2009:150.)

1. ______________________________
2. ______________________________
3. ______________________________
4. ______________________________
5. ______________________________
6. ______________________________
7. ______________________________
8. ______________________________

LABELING EXERCISE 5-10: ENDOCRINE SYSTEM (text Fig. 5-10)

Use different colors to write the names of the numbered structures on the corresponding lines below. Color those same structures within the diagram the corresponding color. Some structures are present in more than one location. Color all of a particular structure the appropriate color. For instance, color or outline all three parathyroid glands, although only one is numbered.

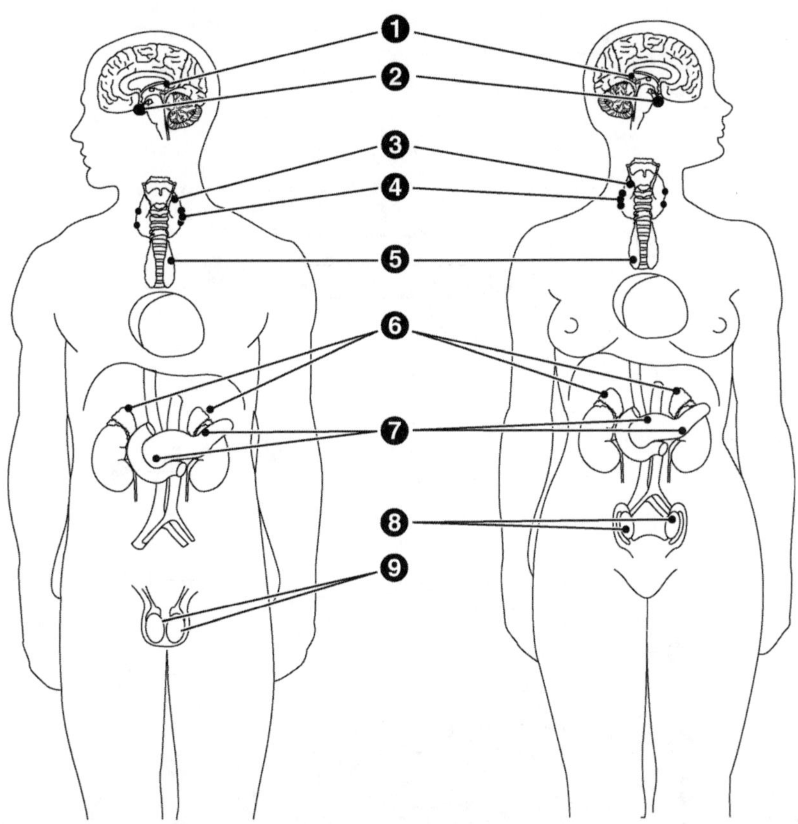

(Adapted with permission from BJ Cohen, KL Hull. *Study Guide for Memmler's the Human Body in Health and Disease,* 11th ed. Philadelphia: Lippincott Williams & Wilkins; 2009:203.)

1. ______________________
2. ______________________
3. ______________________
4. ______________________
5. ______________________
6. ______________________
7. ______________________
8. ______________________
9. ______________________

LABELING EXERCISE 5-11: DIGESTIVE SYSTEM (text Fig. 5-11)

Trace the path of food through the digestive tract by writing the names of the structures numbered 1 through 12 on the corresponding lines. Color all of these structures orange. Then write the names of the accessory organs and ducts on the appropriate lines in different colors. Use black for structure 18. Finally, color the accessory organs with the color used to write their names.

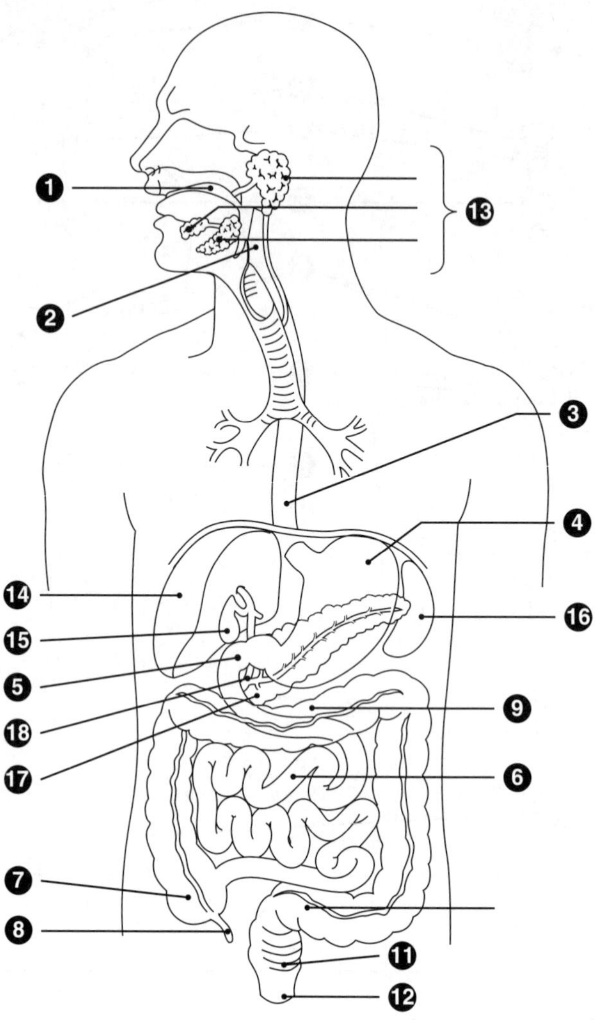

(Adapted with permission from BJ Cohen, KL Hull. *Study Guide for Memmler's the Human Body in Health and Disease*, 11th ed. Philadelphia: Lippincott Williams & Wilkins; 2009:316.)

1. ______________________
2. ______________________
3. ______________________
4. ______________________
5. ______________________
6. ______________________
7. ______________________
8. ______________________
9. ______________________
10. ______________________
11. ______________________
12. ______________________
13. ______________________
14. ______________________
15. ______________________
16. ______________________
17. ______________________
18. ______________________

LABELING EXERCISE 5-12: REPRODUCTIVE SYSTEM (text Fig. 5-12)

Write the names of the numbered structures of the male and female reproductive systems in different colors on the corresponding lines below. Use the same color for structures 1 and 12. Color the structures within the diagrams the colors used to write their names.

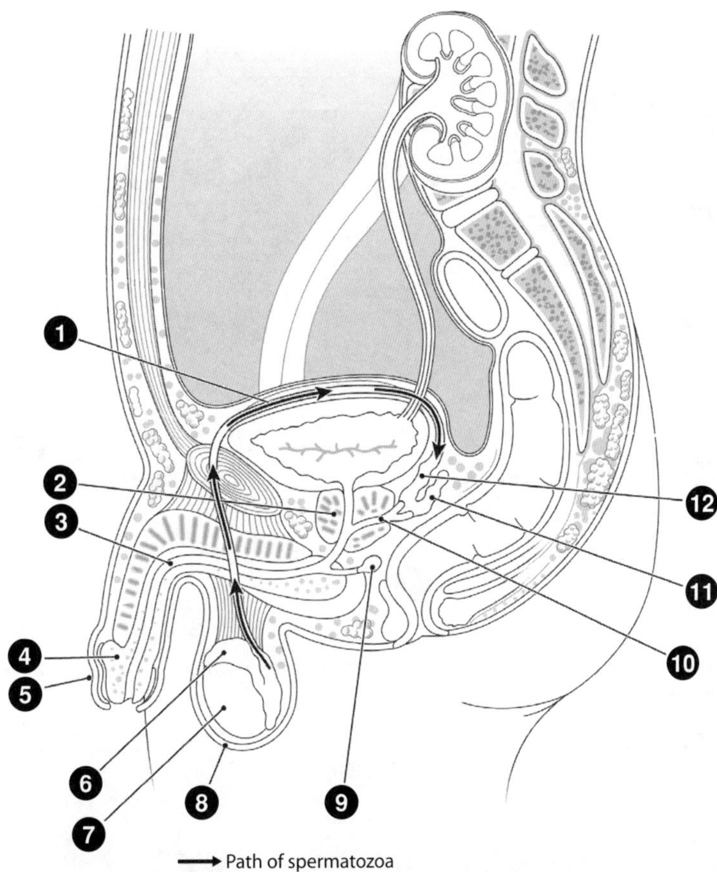

(Adapted with permission from BJ Cohen, KL Hull. *Study Guide for Memmler's the Human Body in Health and Disease,* 11th ed. Philadelphia: Lippincott Williams & Wilkins; 2009:379.)

Male Reproductive System

1. ______________________
2. ______________________
3. ______________________
4. ______________________
5. ______________________
6. ______________________
7. ______________________
8. ______________________
9. ______________________
10. ______________________
11. ______________________
12. ______________________

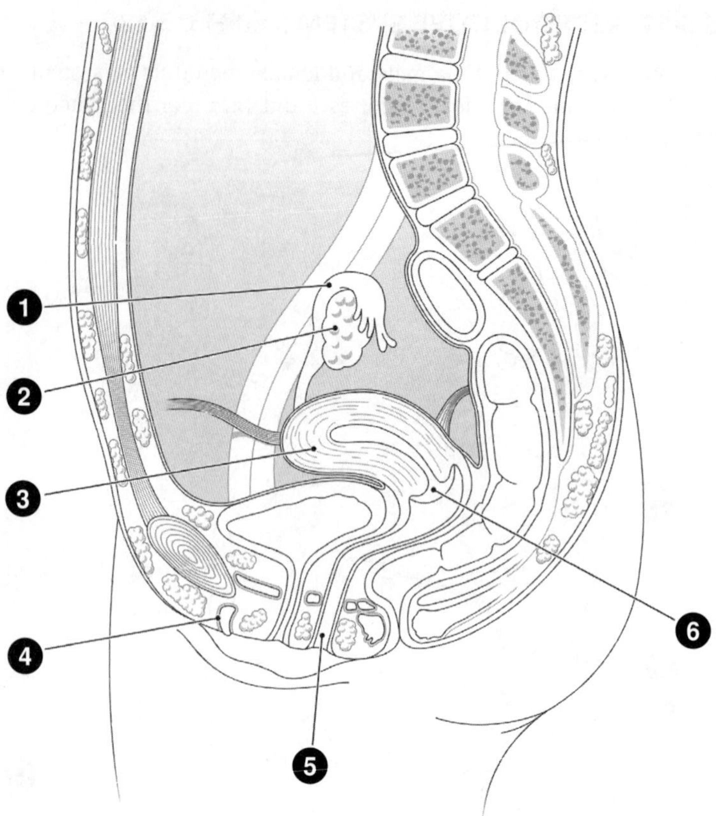

(Adapted with permission from BJ Cohen, KL Hull. *Study Guide for Memmler's the Human Body in Health and Disease*, 11th ed. Philadelphia: Lippincott Williams & Wilkins; 2009: 379, 382.)

Female Reproductive System

1. ___________________________
2. ___________________________
3. ___________________________
4. ___________________________
5. ___________________________
6. ___________________________

LABELING EXERCISE 5-13: URINARY SYSTEM (MALE) (Text Fig. 5-13)

Write the names of the numbered structures on the corresponding lines below. Write the names in different colors using red for arteries and blue for veins. Color the structures within the diagram colors used to write the names. Write the name of the functional unit of the kidney on line 8. Write the name of the filtering tufts of capillaries within the kidney on line 9.

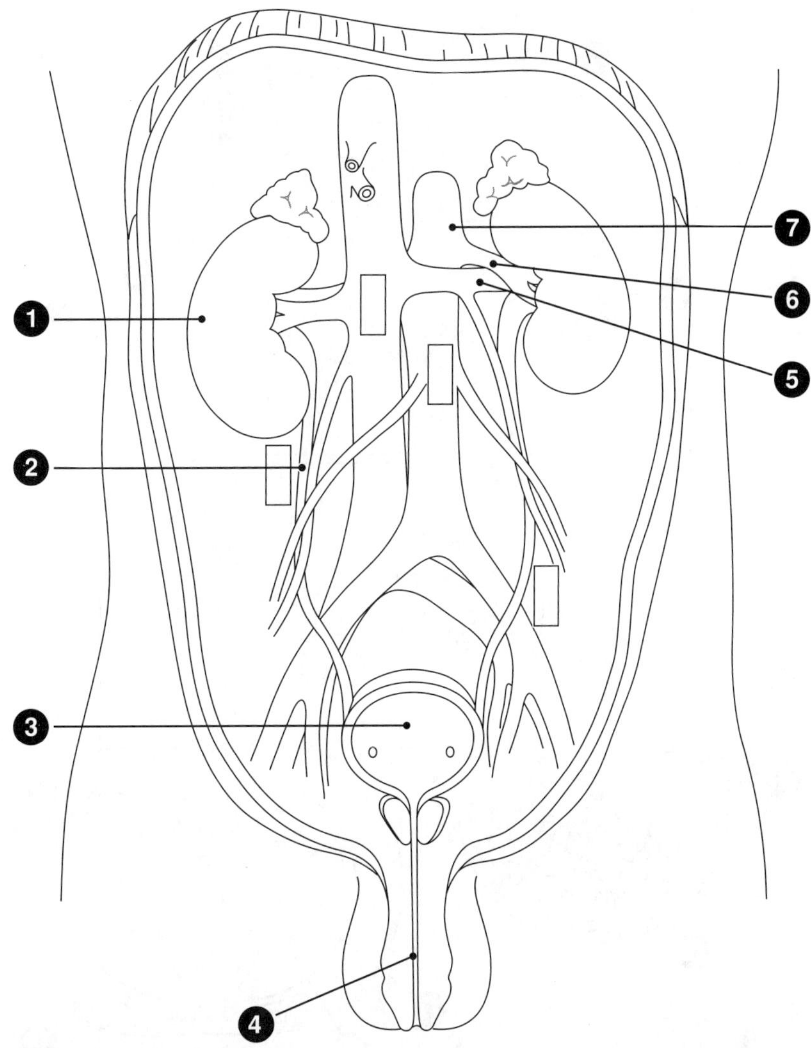

(Adapted with permission from BJ Cohen, KL Hull. *Study Guide for Memmler's the Human Body in Health and Disease,* 11th ed. Philadelphia: Lippincott Williams & Wilkins; 2009:356.)

1. ______________________

2. ______________________

3. ______________________

4. ______________________

5. ______________________

6. ______________________

7. ______________________

8. ______________________

9. ______________________

LABELING EXERCISE 5-14: RESPIRATORY SYSTEM (text Fig. 5-14)

Write the names of the numbered structures on the corresponding lines below (see figure on the following page). Then use green to color all of the structures that encounter inspired air.

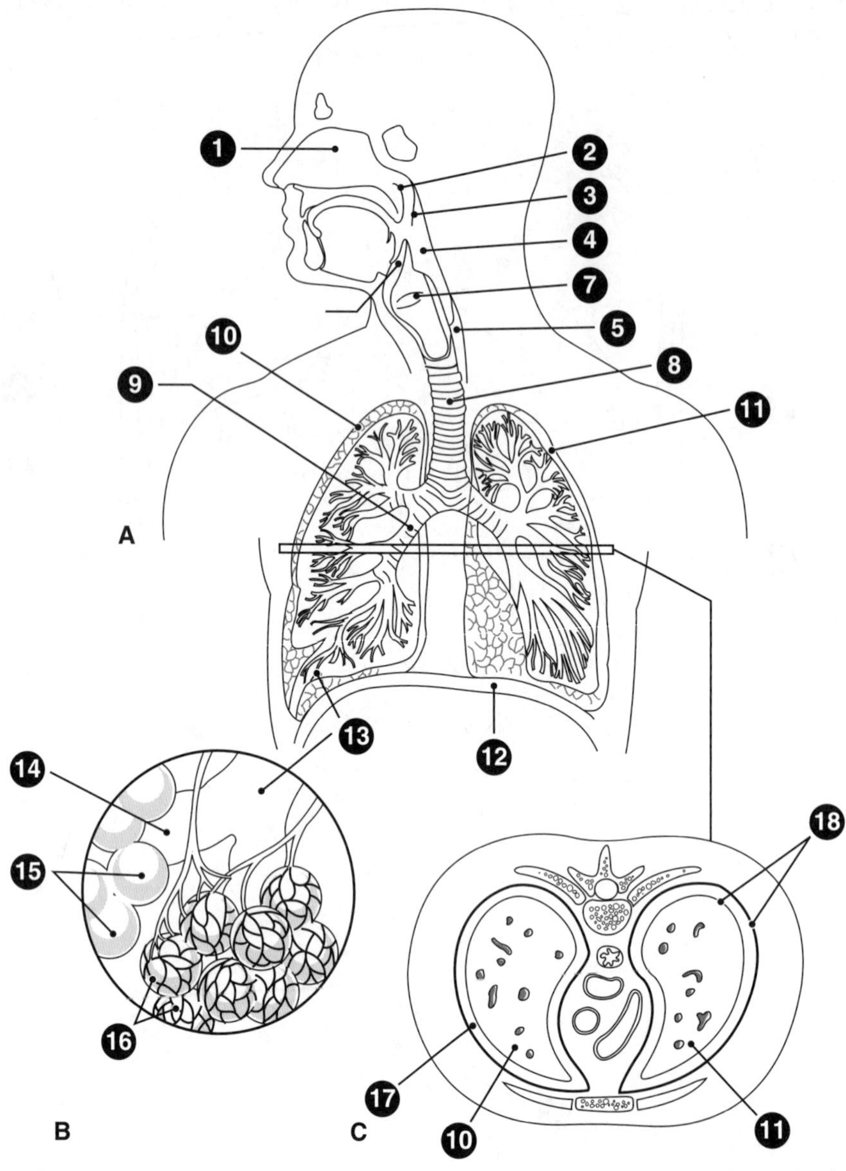

(Adapted with permission from BJ Cohen, KL Hull. *Study Guide for Memmler's the Human Body in Health and Disease*, 11th ed. Philadelphia: Lippincott Williams & Wilkins; 2009:298.)

1. ______________________
2. ______________________
3. ______________________
4. ______________________
5. ______________________
6. ______________________
7. ______________________
8. ______________________
9. ______________________
10. ______________________
11. ______________________
12. ______________________
13. ______________________
14. ______________________
15. ______________________
16. ______________________
17. ______________________
18. ______________________

Knowledge Drills

KNOWLEDGE DRILL 5-1: KEY POINT RECOGNITION

The following sentences are taken from Key Point statements found in Chapter 5 of the textbook. Fill in the blanks with the missing information.

1. Blood Creatine is a measure of kidney function because (A) ____________ is a (B) ____________ product normally removed from the blood by the (C) ____________.
2. Pregnancy tests are based on a reaction with a hormone called (A) ____________ ____________ ____________ secreted by (B) ____________ cells that eventually give rise to the (C) ____________.
3. (A) ____________ terms are relative positions in respect to other parts of the body. For example, the ankle can be described as (B) ____________ to the leg and (C) ____________ to the foot.
4. Bones of particular importance in blood collection are the distal (A) ____________ of the (B) ____________ and the (C) ____________ or (D) ____________ bone of the foot.
5. A deficiency of (A) ____________ in premature infants causes the (B) ____________ to collapse leading to a condition called (C) ____________ ____________ ____________ ____________.
6. When a typical cell duplicates itself, the (A) ____________ doubles and the cell (B) ____________ by a process called (C) ____________.
7. Skeletal muscle (A) ____________ helps keep blood moving through your (B) ____________. For example, moving your (C) ____________ helps move blood from your fingertips back to your (D) ____________.
8. The (A) ____________ cavity is separated from the (B) ____________ cavity by a muscle called the (C) ____________.

KNOWLEDGE DRILL 5-2: SCRAMBLED WORDS

Instructions: Unscramble the following words using the hints given in parenthesis. Write the correct spelling of the scrambled word on the line next to it.

1. tralenxe EXTERNAL (near the surface)
2. blosmania ANABOLISM (constructive process)
3. ratgelaic CARTILLAGE (connective tissue)
4. haxplan PHALANX (a short bone)
5. lekestla SKELETAL (type of muscle)
6. clanugo GLUCAGON (stimulates the liver)
7. gemsenin MENEGIES (a problem if inflamed)
8. yasleam AMYLASE (aids in digestion)
9. tageem GAMETE (could end up a human)
10. tranufscat SURFACTANT (lungs need it)

Skills Drills

SKILLS DRILL 5-1: REQUISITION ACTIVITY

Any Hospital USA
1123 West Physician Drive
Any Town USA

Laboratory Test Requisition

PATIENT INFORMATION:

Name: Doe (last) John (first) C (MI) DOB: 12-05-52

Identification Number: 0673519285 Location: 302B

Referring Physician: Martinez

Date to be Collected: 05/09/2011 Time to be Collected: 0600

Special Instructions: fasting

TEST(S) REQUIRED:

____ NH4 – Ammonia	____ Hgb – hemoglobin
____ Bili – Bilirubin, total & direct	____ Lact – lactic acid/lactate
____ BMP – basic metabolic panel	X Lytes – electrolytes
____ BUN – Blood urea nitrogen	____ Plt. Ct. – platelet count
____ CBC – complete blood count	X PSA – prostate specific antigen
X Chol – cholesterol	____ PT – prothrombin time
____ D–dimer	____ PTT – partial thromboplastin time
____ ESR – erythrocyte sed rate	____ RPR – rapid plasma reagin
____ ETOH – alcohol	X UA – Urinalysis
____ Gluc – glucose	Other TSH & Uric Acid

Identify one body system associated with each of the tests ordered on the requisition below. Write the test abbreviations (if applicable) and the associated body systems on the following lines in the order the tests appear on the requisition starting with the left column.

1. DIGESTIVE
2. URINARY / RESPIRATORY
3. REPRODUCTIVE
4. URINARY
5. ENDOCINE
6. SKELETAL

SKILLS DRILL 5-2: WORD BUILDING

Divide each word into all of its elements: preface (P), word root (WR), combining vowel (CV), and suffix (S). Write the word part, its definition, and the general meaning of the word on the corresponding lines. If the word does not have a particular word part, write NA (not applicable) in its place.

Example: hyperglycemia

Elements *hyper* / *glyc* / ____ / *emia*
P WR CV S

Definitions *too much* / *glucose* / ____ / *blood condition*

Meaning: a condition in which the blood sugar/glucose is high

1. Osteochondritis

Elements ____________ / ____________ / ____ / ____________
P WR CV S

Definitions ____________ / ____________ / ____ / ____________

Meaning:

2. Electromyogram ____________ / ____________ / ____ / ____________
P WR CV S

Definitions ____________ / ____________ / ____ / ____________

Meaning:

3. Physiology ____________ / ____________ / ____ / ____________
P WR CV S

Definitions ____________ / ____________ / ____ / ____________

Meaning:

4. Thrombophlebitis ____________ / ____________ / ____ / ____________
P WR CV S

Definitions ____________ / ____________ / ____ / ____________

Meaning:

5. Dermatitis ____________ / ____________ / ____ / ____________
P WR CV S

Definitions ____________ / ____________ / ____ / ____________

Meaning:

6. Arthritis ____________ / ____________ / ____ / ____________
P WR CV S

Definitions ____________ / ____________ / ____ / ____________

Meaning:

Crossword

ACROSS

1. Act of turning the palm up
4. Small synovial-fluid-filled sacs near joints
6. O_2 and CO_2 form when disassociated from hgb
7. Farthest from center of the body or point of attachment
8. Science of the functions of living organisms
10. Threadlike fiber carrying messages away from a nerve cell
11. Glands that secrete substances through ducts
13. Lateral, forearm bone
14. Sex cells
17. True skin
20. Medial forearm bone
21. Female reproductive gland containing ova
22. Large medial bone of the leg below the knee
23. Fundamental working unit of the nervous system
24. Aggregate of similar cells or types of cells
25. Multiple sclerosis (abbrev.)
26. Arterial blood gas procedure (abbrev.)
27. Dense connective tissue that makes up the skeletal system (pl.)
30. Concerning the palm of the hand
31. Intravenous pyelography (abbrev.)
33. Digestive system disorder that exhibits as a lesion
34. Largest accessory organ in the digestive system
36. A chronic lung disorder where exhaled air is obstructed (abbrev.)
37. Pancreatic disorder involving insulin
38. Nonliving material primarily composed of keratin

DOWN

1. Plane dividing the body into right and left portions
2. Nervous system division serving the body periphery (abbrev.)
3. Convoluted tubular structure in the kidney
4. Material part of a human described as head, neck, trunk, and limbs
5. Body process that converts simple compounds to complex substances
9. Substance that coats the wall of alveoli
12. Outside the blood vessels
15. Fibrous tissue that replaces normal tissue destroyed by injury
16. Hormone secreted by beta cells in the islets of Langerhans
18. Female hormone that stimulates secondary sex characteristics
19. Broad, flaring portion of the hip bone
26. Gland on top of each kidney
27. Fluid secreted by the liver that aids digestion of fat
28. Test that monitors joint swelling (abbrev.)
29. Bean-shaped organ located at the back of abdominal cavity
32. Test used to diagnose cervical cancer
35. Test that records brain waves (abbrev.)

Chapter Review Questions

1. The functional units of the nervous system are the
   a. axons.
   b. dendrites.
   c. nephrons.
   d. neurons.

2. A person who is supine is
   a. lying face up.
   b. lying on the side.
   c. sitting up.
   d. standing erect.

3. The creation of a hormone is an example of
   a. anabolism.
   b. catabolism.
   c. hemopoiesis.
   d. homeostasis.

4. Which of the following is a structure within a cell?
   a. Alveolus
   b. Glomerulus
   c. Golgi apparatus
   d. Pharynx

5. Which of the following is a finger bone?
   a. Calcaneus
   b. Phalanx
   c. Tarsal
   d. Tibia

6. Which of the following is an appendage of the integumentary system?
   a. Adrenal gland
   b. Pineal gland
   c. Sebaceous gland
   d. Thymus gland

7. A patient has meningitis. What body system is associated with this diagnosis?
   a. Digestive
   b. Endocrine
   c. Nervous
   d. Urinary

8. Which of the following are urinary system structures?
   a. Meninges
   b. Glomeruli
   c. Islets of Langerhans
   d. Papillae

9. Accessory organs of the digestive system include
   a. the gallbladder.
   b. the liver.
   c. the pancreas.
   d. all of the above.

10. Which of the following are all endocrine system tests?
    a. ABGs, CBC, lytes
    b. CBC, ESR, uric acid
    c. FSH, HCG, RPR
    d. T_3, T_4, TSH

11. Most carbon dioxide is carried in the blood in this manner.
    a. As bicarbonate ion
    b. As Pco_2
    c. Bound to hemoglobin
    d. Dissolved in the blood plasma

12. You are looking at muscle tissue under the microscope. The cells you see are long, cylindrical, multinucleated, and heavily striated. What type of muscle cells are they?
    a. Cardiac
    b. Involuntary
    c. Smooth
    d. Skeletal

13. Gametes are
    a. blood-filtering structures.
    b. cytoplasmic organelles.
    c. dermal structures.
    d. sex cells.

14. Surfactant
    a. helps keep alveoli inflated.
    b. is secreted by sebaceous glands.
    c. is a digestive enzyme.
    d. lubricates joints.

15. Which of the following tests is associated with the reproductive system?
    a. ABG
    b. HCG
    c. O&P
    d. UA

CASE STUDIES

Case Study 5-1 Body Systems, Disorders, and Directional Terms

An older female outpatient arrives for a blood draw. The tests requested include ESR and estrogen levels. The patient walks in very slowly, as if her joints were stiff or sore. She has an oxygen tank with her. By the time she sits down in the chair, she is out of breath. When the phlebotomist attempts to locate a vein for the blood draw, the patient can only partly straighten her right arm and indicates that it is too painful to straighten it any further. The patient says that she cannot be drawn in the other arm because she has had a mastectomy on that side. The phlebotomist chooses a prominent vein on the medial aspect of the ventral surface of the arm slightly distal to the bend in the elbow to perform the blood draw.

QUESTIONS

1. Which of the patient's body systems are being evaluated at this time? ENDOCIRINE SYSTEM
2. Name several disorders the patient could have based on her symptoms. COPD, ARTHRITIS, MYALGIA, ATROP
3. Where did the phlebotomist collect the specimen?
   RIGHT ARM INSIDE AT THE FOREARM

Case Study 5-2 Body Systems, Disorders, Diagnostic Tests, and Directional Terms

A phlebotomist is called to the ER to collect ABGs on a patient. The patient is highly agitated and hyperventilating. The phlebotomist collects the ABG specimen from an artery on the lateral aspect of the left ventral wrist proximal to the crease in the wrist.

QUESTIONS

1. What does the abbreviation ABG stand for?
   ARTIRIAL BLOOD GASES
2. What body system is evaluated with the ABG test?
   RESPIRATORY
3. What effect does hyperventilation have on CO_2 levels and pH? IMBALANCE OF CO_2
4. What dangerous condition can hyperventilation cause? FAINTING
5. Where did the phlebotomist collect the specimen?
   LATERAL SIDE WHERE THE WRIST MEETS THE FOREARM.

CHAPTER

6

The Circulatory System

OBJECTIVES

Study the information in your textbook that corresponds to each objective to prepare yourself for the activities in this chapter.

1. Define the key terms and abbreviations listed at the beginning of this chapter.
2. Identify the layers and other structures of the heart and describe their function.
3. Describe the cardiac cycle and how an ECG tracing relates to it; explain the origins of heart sounds and pulse rates.
4. Describe how to take blood pressure readings and what they represent.
5. Identify the two main divisions of the vascular system, describe the function of each, and trace the flow of blood throughout the system.
6. Identify the different types of blood vessels and describe the structure and function of each.
7. Name and locate major arm and leg veins and describe the suitability of each for venipuncture.
8. List the major constituents of blood, describe the function of each of the formed elements, and differentiate between serum, plasma, and whole blood.
9. Describe how ABO and Rh blood types are determined and the importance of compatibility testing before transfusion.
10. Define hemostasis and describe basic coagulation and fibrinolysis processes.
11. Identify the structures and vessels of the lymphatic system and describe their function.
12. List the disorders and diagnostic tests of the circulatory system.

Matching

Use choices only once unless otherwise indicated.

MATCHING 6-1: KEY TERMS AND DESCRIPTIONS

Match the key term with the *best* description.

Key Terms (1–14)

1. _____ antecubital
2. _____ arrhythmia
3. _____ atria
4. _____ basilic vein
5. _____ blood pressure
6. _____ cardiac cycle
7. _____ cephalic vein
8. _____ coagulation
9. _____ cross-match
10. _____ diastole
11. _____ ECG/EKG
12. _____ erythrocyte
13. _____ extrinsic
14. _____ fibrinolysis

Descriptions (1–14)

A. Antecubital vein in the lateral aspect of the arm
B. Blood-clotting process
C. Force exerted by the blood on the walls of the blood vessels
D. Irregularity in the heart rate, rhythm, or beat
E. Large antecubital vein on the inner side of the arm
F. Medical term for red blood cell (RBC)
G. Medical term meaning in front of the elbow
H. One complete contraction and subsequent relaxation of the heart
I. Originating outside
J. Process that leads to dissolution of a blood clot
K. Record of the electrical activity of the heart
L. Relaxing phase of the cardiac cycle
M. Test to determine compatibility of blood for transfusion
N. Upper, receiving chambers of the heart

Key Terms (15–28)

15. _____ hemostasis
16. _____ intrinsic
17. _____ leukocyte
18. _____ median cubital vein
19. _____ plasma
20. _____ pulmonary circulation
21. _____ serum
22. _____ sphygmomanometer
23. _____ systemic circulation
24. _____ systole
25. _____ thrombin
26. _____ thrombocyte
27. _____ vasoconstriction
28. _____ ventricles

Descriptions (15–28)

A. Blood pressure cuff
B. Contracting phase of the cardiac cycle
C. Fluid portion of clotted blood
D. Fluid portion of whole blood
E. Lower chambers of the heart, which deliver blood to the arteries
F. Main coagulation enzyme
G. Medical term for platelet
H. Medical term for white blood cell (WBC)
I. Originating within
J. Process by which the body stops blood loss after injury
K. Reduction in blood vessel diameter due to contraction of tunica media muscles
L. System that carries blood from the heart to the body tissues and back
M. System that carries blood from the heart to the lungs and back
N. Vein located near the middle of the antecubital fossa area

MATCHING 6-2: CIRCULATORY SYSTEM STRUCTURES, DISORDERS, AND DIAGNOSTIC TESTS

Match the structures, disorders, and diagnostic tests with the circulatory system components with which they are associated in the textbook.

Structures

1. B atria
2. C axillary node
3. B endocardium
4. A eosinophil
5. D median vein
6. A reticulocyte
7. B septum
8. C thoracic duct
9. B tricuspid valve
10. D tunica media

Disorders

1. A anemia
2. B angina pectoris
3. D atherosclerosis
4. B endocarditis
5. C Hodgkin disease
6. C lymphoma
7. B myocardial infarction
8. D phlebitis
9. A polycythemia
10. A thrombocytopenia

Diagnostic Tests

1. B ABGs
2. C CBC
3. B CK
4. D D-dimer
5. B digoxin
6. A ferritin
7. A Hgb
8. C mono test
9. D PT
10. B troponin T

Circulatory System Components

A. Blood
B. Heart
C. Lymphatic system
D. Vascular system

MATCHING 6-3: HEMOSTATIC RESPONSE AND ACTION

Match the hemostatic response with the correct action. Choices may be used more than once.

Hemostatic Response

A. Vasoconstriction
B. Platelet plug formation
C. Hemostatic plug formation
D. Fibrinolysis

Action

1. _____ amplification
2. _____ blood vessel contraction
3. _____ cross-linkage of fibrin
4. _____ initiation
5. _____ fibrin degradation
6. _____ platelet adhesion
7. _____ propagation
8. _____ soluble fibrin generation
9. _____ thrombin burst
10. _____ tissue factor activation

Labeling Exercises

LABELING EXERCISE 6-1: THE HEART AND GREAT VESSELS (text Fig. 6-1)

Write the name of each numbered structure on the corresponding numbered line. Write the names of hollow spaces and vessels that contain deoxygenated blood in blue and those that contain oxygenated blood in red. Write the names of all other structures in black. Next, color the layers and partition of the heart pink, the valves yellow, the vessels and structures that carry deoxygenated blood blue, and the vessels and structures that carry oxygenated blood red. Finally, draw arrows to indicate the direction of blood flow.

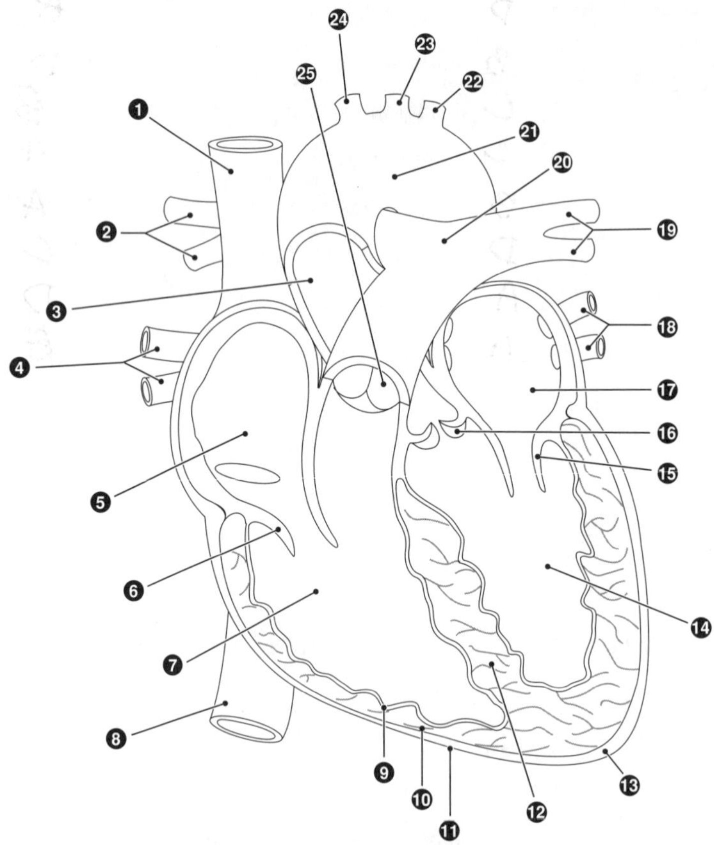

(Adapted with permission from Cohen BJ, Hull KL. *Study Guide for Memmler's the Human Body in Health and Disease,* 11th ed. Philadelphia: Lippincott Williams & Wilkins; 2009:236.)

1. ______________________
2. ______________________
3. ______________________
4. ______________________
5. ______________________
6. ______________________
7. ______________________
8. ______________________
9. ______________________
10. ______________________
11. ______________________
12. ______________________
13. ______________________
14. ______________________
15. ______________________
16. ______________________
17. ______________________
18. ______________________
19. ______________________
20. ______________________
21. ______________________
22. ______________________
23. ______________________
24. ______________________
25. ______________________

LABELING EXERCISE 6-2: ELECTRICAL CONDUCTION SYSTEM OF THE HEART (text Fig. 6-2)

Write the name of each numbered structure of the electrical conduction system on the corresponding numbered line. Write the names of hollow spaces and vessels that contain deoxygenated blood in blue and those that contain oxygenated blood in red. Next, color the structures that conduct electrical impulses yellow. Color the vessels and structures that carry deoxygenated blood blue and those that carry oxygenated blood red. Finally, place a star on the drawing next to the number of the structure that originates the electrical impulse.

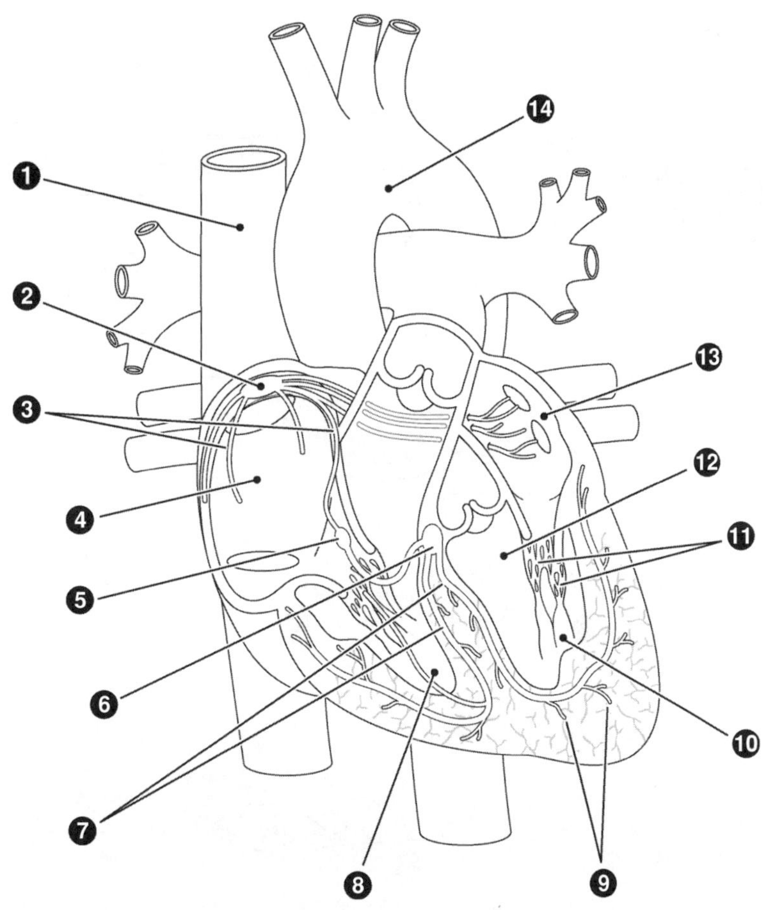

(Adapted with permission from Cohen BJ, Hull KL. *Study Guide for Memmler's the Human Body in Health and Disease,* 11th ed. Philadelphia: Lippincott Williams & Wilkins; 2009:238.)

1. ______________________
2. ______________________
3. ______________________
4. ______________________
5. ______________________
6. ______________________
7. ______________________
8. ______________________
9. ______________________
10. ______________________
11. ______________________
12. ______________________
13. ______________________
14. ______________________

LABELING EXERCISE 6-3: ARTERY, VEIN, AND CAPILLARY STRUCTURE (text Fig. 6-8)

Write the names of the vessel types labeled 1 through 5 on the corresponding numbered line, writing the name in red if the vessel carries arterial blood, blue if the vessel carries venous blood, and purple if the vessel carries a mixture of both. Then, write the names of the vascular layers labeled 6 to 10 on the corresponding numbered line. Next, color the single-layered blood vessel and the inside of the large blood vessels pink. Color the outside layer of structures that carry arterial blood red and the outside of the structures that carry venous blood blue. Finally, draw an arrow in the box to represent the direction of blood flow.

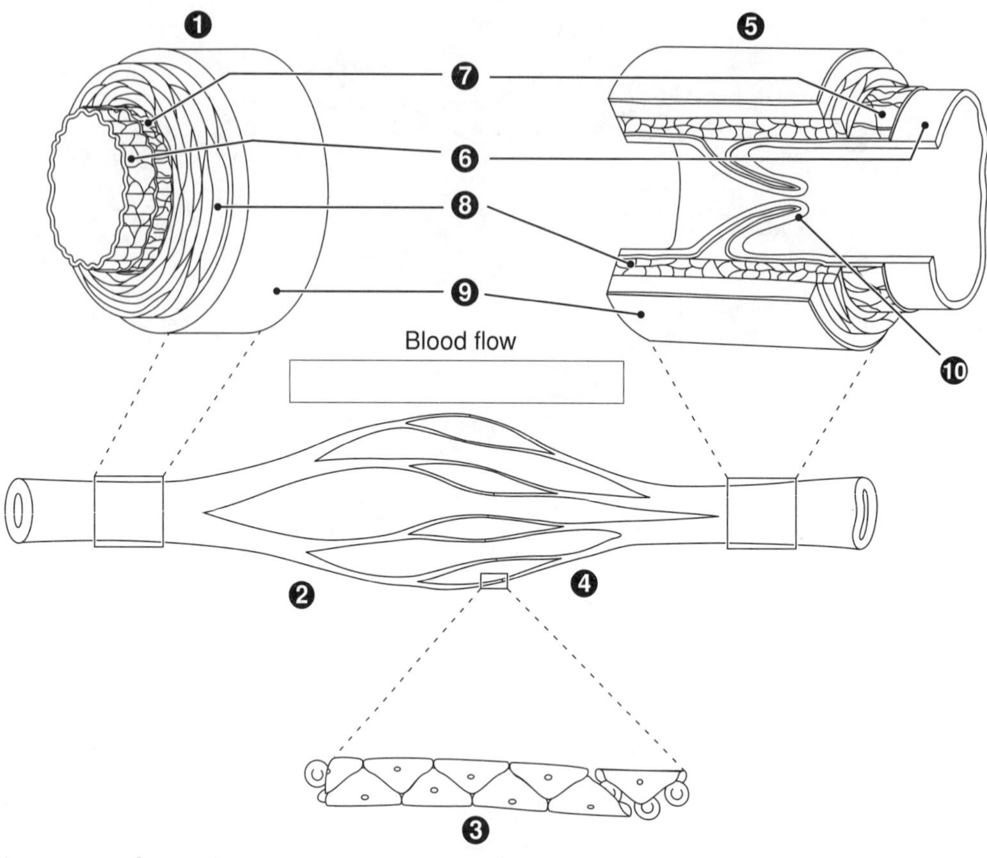

(Adapted with permission from Cohen BJ, Hull KL. *Study Guide for Memmler's the Human Body in Health and Disease*, 11th ed. Philadelphia: Lippincott Williams & Wilkins; 2009:249.)

1. ______________________
2. ______________________
3. ______________________
4. ______________________
5. ______________________
6. ______________________
7. ______________________
8. ______________________
9. ______________________
10. ______________________

LABELING EXERCISE 6-4: REPRESENTATION OF THE VASCULAR FLOW (text Fig. 6-10)

Write the name of each numbered structure or tissue on the corresponding numbered line. Next, color deoxygenated blood flow blue and oxygenated blood flow red. Then draw arrows to show the direction of blood flow.

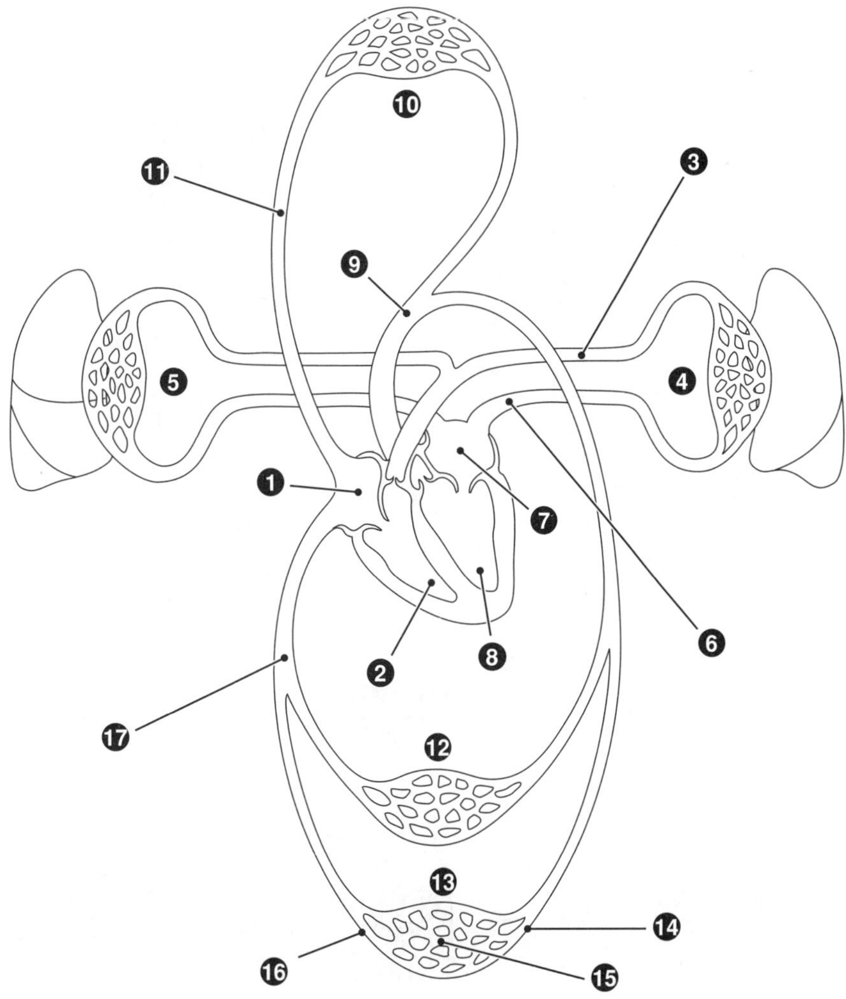

(Adapted with permission from Cohen BJ, Hull KL. *Study Guide for Memmler's the Human Body in Health and Disease,* 11th ed. Philadelphia: Lippincott Williams & Wilkins; 2009:235.)

1. ______________________
2. ______________________
3. ______________________
4. ______________________
5. ______________________
6. ______________________
7. ______________________
8. ______________________
9. ______________________
10. ______________________
11. ______________________
12. ______________________
13. ______________________
14. ______________________
15. ______________________
16. ______________________
17. ______________________

LABELING EXERCISE 6-5: ARM AND HAND VEINS (text Fig. 6-11)

Write the name of each numbered structure on the corresponding numbered line.

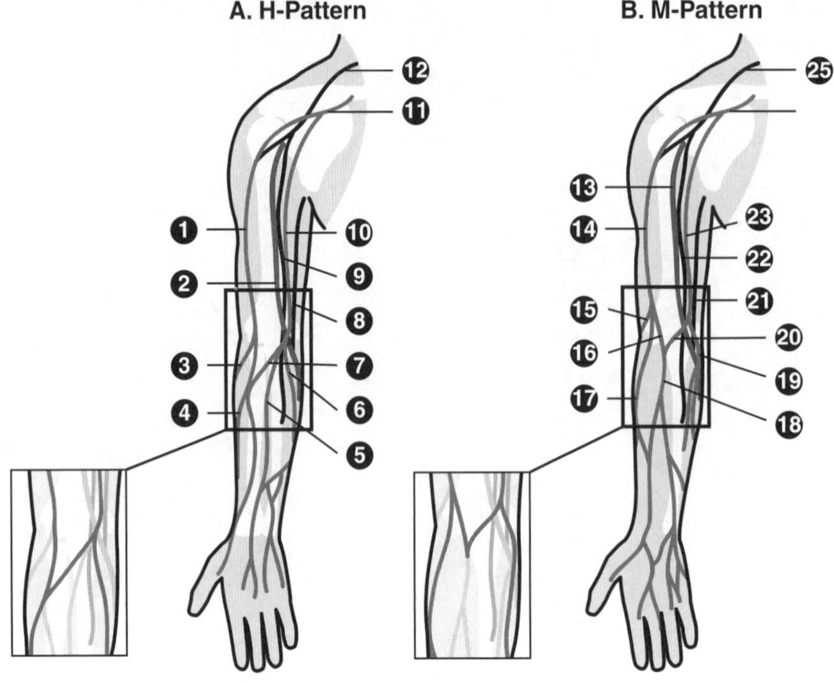

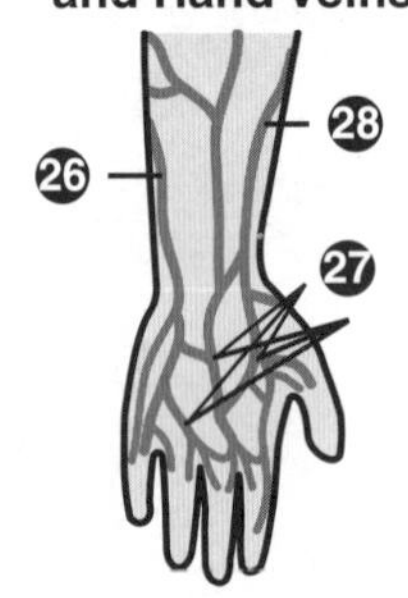

1. __________
2. __________
3. __________
4. __________
5. __________
6. __________
7. __________
8. __________
9. __________
10. __________
11. __________
12. __________
13. __________
14. __________
15. __________
16. __________
17. __________
18. __________
19. __________
20. __________
21. __________
22. __________
23. __________
24. __________
25. __________
26. __________
27. __________
28. __________

LABELING EXERCISE 6-6: LEG VEINS (text Fig. 6-12)

Write the name of each numbered structure on the corresponding numbered line.

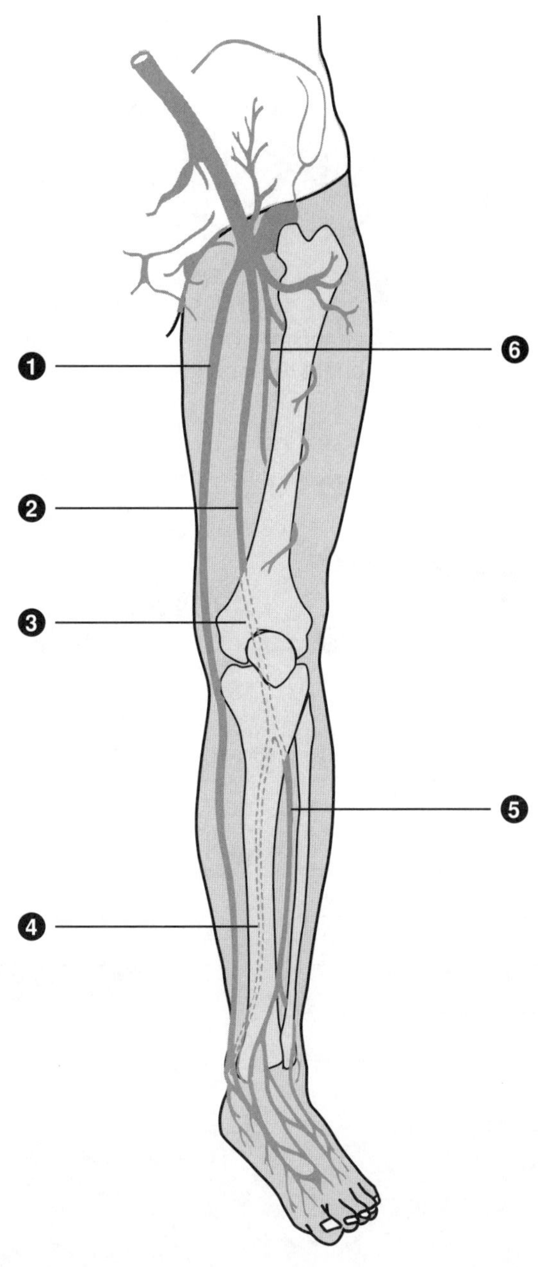

1. ______________________
2. ______________________
3. ______________________
4. ______________________
5. ______________________
6. ______________________

LABELING EXERCISE 6-7: BLOOD CELLS (text Figs. 6-15 and 6-16)

Write the names of the types of leukocytes identified by the numbers 1 through 5 on the corresponding numbered lines. Then write the names of the cells or cell parts identified by numbers 6 through 9 on the corresponding numbered line.

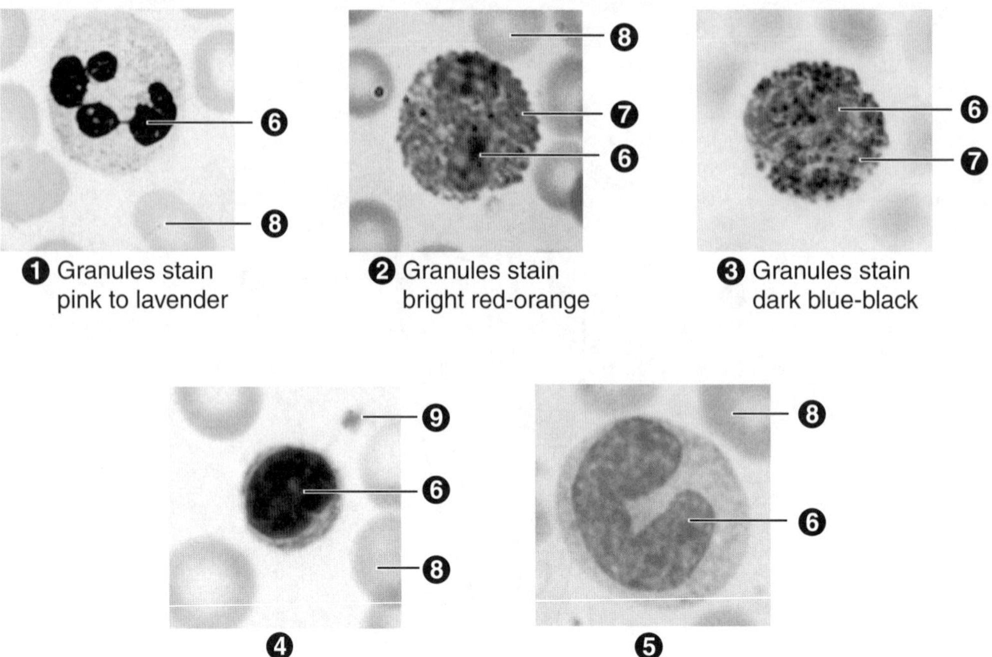

(Adapted with permission from Cohen BJ, Hull KL. *Study Guide for Memmler's the Human Body in Health and Disease,* 11th ed. Philadelphia: Lippincott Williams & Wilkins; 2009:219.)

1. ______________________
2. ______________________
3. ______________________
4. ______________________
5. ______________________
6. ______________________
7. ______________________
8. ______________________
9. ______________________

LABELING EXERCISE 6-8: CENTRIFUGED WHOLE-BLOOD SPECIMEN (text Fig. 6-18)

Write the names of the specimen parts identified by numbers 1 through 3 on the corresponding numbered line.

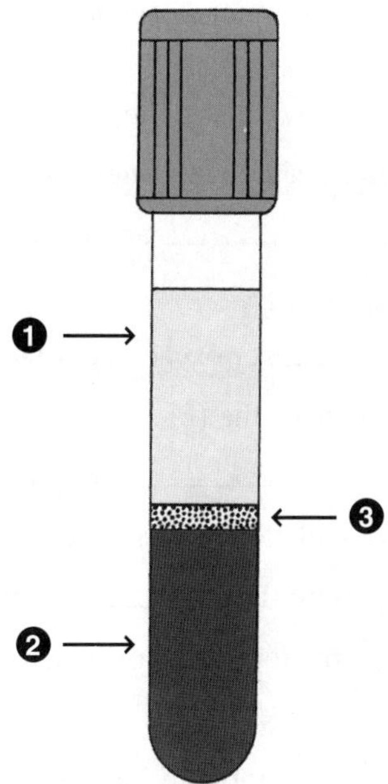

1. ______________________________
2. ______________________________
3. ______________________________

Knowledge Drills

KNOWLEDGE DRILL 6-1: CAUTION AND KEY POINT RECOGNITION

The following sentences have been taken from caution and key point statements found throughout Chapter 6. Fill in the blanks with the missing information.

1. Vein (A) __________ differs somewhat from person to person and you may not see the exact textbook pattern. The important thing to remember is to choose a (B)__________ vein that is well fixed and does not overlie a (C) __________, which indicates the presence of an (D) __________ and the potential presence of a major (E) __________.
2. The (A) __________ artery is the only artery that carries (B) __________, or oxygen-poor blood. It is part of the (C) __________ circulation and carries (D) __________ blood from the (E) __________ to the (F) __________. It is classified as an artery because it carries blood (G) __________ from the heart.
3. The natural (A) __________ circulate in the plasma along with the coagulation factors. They keep the (B) __________ process in check and limited to (C) __________ sites by (D) __________ (breaking down) any (E) __________ coagulation factors that (F) __________ the injury site or remain within the formed clot.
4. When (A) __________ blood is collected by syringe, the (B) __________ normally causes the blood to (C) __________ or __________ into the syringe under its own (D) __________.
5. Veins on the (A) __________ of the (B) __________ are never (C) __________ for venipuncture.
6. A (A) __________ (BT) test assesses (B) __________ formation in the (C) __________.
7. The presence of (A) __________ within (B) __________ is a major (C) __________ difference between arteries and veins.
8. Testing personnel typically prefer specimens that contain roughly (A) __________ times the amount of sample required to perform the test; so the test can be (B) __________ if needed with some to spare. Consequently, a test that requires 1 mL of (C) __________ or plasma would require a (D) __________ blood specimen because only half the specimen will be (E) __________, while a test that requires 1 mL (F) __________ blood would require a (G) __________ specimen.
9. (A) __________ lymph nodes (nodes in the armpit) are often removed as part of (B)__________ cancer surgery. Their removal can impair (c) __________ drainage and interfere with the destruction of (D) __________ and foreign matter. This is cause for concern in phlebotomy and the reason an (E) __________ on the same side as a (F) __________ is not suitable for venipuncture.
10. The main component of RBCs is (A) __________ an (B) __________ containing pigment that enables them to transport (C) __________ and (D) __________ and also gives them their (E) __________.

KNOWLEDGE DRILL 6-2: SCRAMBLED WORDS

Unscramble the following words using the hints given in parenthesis. Write the correct spelling of the scrambled word on the line next to it.

1. shenioda ______________________ (a platelet function)
2. gingatulitano ______________________ (a transfusion worry)
3. sidelota ______________________ (part of the cardiac cycle)
4. philamihoe ______________________ (coagulation disorder)
5. yomplahm ______________________ (lymphatic system disorder)
6. pichlace ______________________ (a safe vein choice)
7. daymirmuco ______________________ (the muscle behind the “pump”)
8. nopulamrechlorpoy ______________________ (describes a type of WBC)
9. nesmulria ______________________ (like a half-moon)
10. critsovonnastico ______________________ (helps prevent blood loss)

Skills Drills

SKILLS DRILL 6-1: REQUISITION ACTIVITY

You have received the following test order. Name the circulatory system part or process associated with each test ordered. Write the answer in the margin next to the test.

Any Hospital USA
1123 West Physician Drive
Any Town USA

Laboratory Test Requisition

PATIENT INFORMATION:

Name: Doe (last) Jane (first) M (MI)

Identification Number: 03265791 Birth Date: 09/17/55

Referring Physician: Goodhart

Date to be Collected: 06/22/11 Time to be Collected: 0600

Special Instructions: Patient is on a blood thinner

TEST(S) REQUIRED:

____ NH4 – Ammonia	____ Gluc – glucose
____ Bili – Bilirubin, total & direct	X Hgb – hemoglobin BLOOD
____ BMP – basic metabolic panel	____ Lact – lactic acid/lactate
____ BUN - Blood urea nitrogen	____ Plt. Ct. – platelet count
____ Lytes – electrolytes	X PT – prothrombin time - VASCULAR
____ CBC – complete blood count	____ PTT – partial thromboplastin time
HEART X Chol – cholesterol	____ RPR – rapid plasma reagin
____ ESR – erythrocyte sed rate	____ T&S – type and screen
____ EtOH - alcohol	____ PSA – prostatic specific antigen
____ D-dime	X Other Digoxin - HEART

SKILLS DRILL 6-2: WORD BUILDING

Divide each word into all of its elements (parts): prefix (P), word root (WR), combining vowel (CV), and suffix (S). Write the word part, its definition, and the meaning of the word on the corresponding lines. If the word does not have a particular element, write NA (not applicable) in its place.

Example: Pericardium

Elements _*peri*_ / _*card*_ / ___ / _*ium*_
P WR CV S

Definitions _*around*_ / _*heart*_ / ___ / _*structure*_

Meaning: structure around the heart

1. Erythrocyte

Elements ______ / ______ / ___ / ______
P WR CV S

Definitions ______ / ______ / ___ / ______

Meaning:

2. Anemia

Elements ______ / ______ / ___ / ______
P WR CV S

Definitions ______ / ______ / ___ / ______

Meaning:

3. Hemostatic

Elements ______ / ______ / ___ / ______
P WR CV S

Definitions ______ / ______ / ___ / ______

Meaning:

4. Endocarditis

Elements ______ / ______ / ___ / ______
P WR CV S

Definitions ______ / ______ / ___ / ______

Meaning:

5. Toxic

Elements ______ / ______ / ___ / ______
P WR CV S

Definitions ______ / ______ / ___ / ______

Meaning:

6. Thrombocyte

Elements ______ / ______ / ___ / ______
P WR CV S

Definitions ______ / ______ / ___ / ______

Meaning:

Crossword

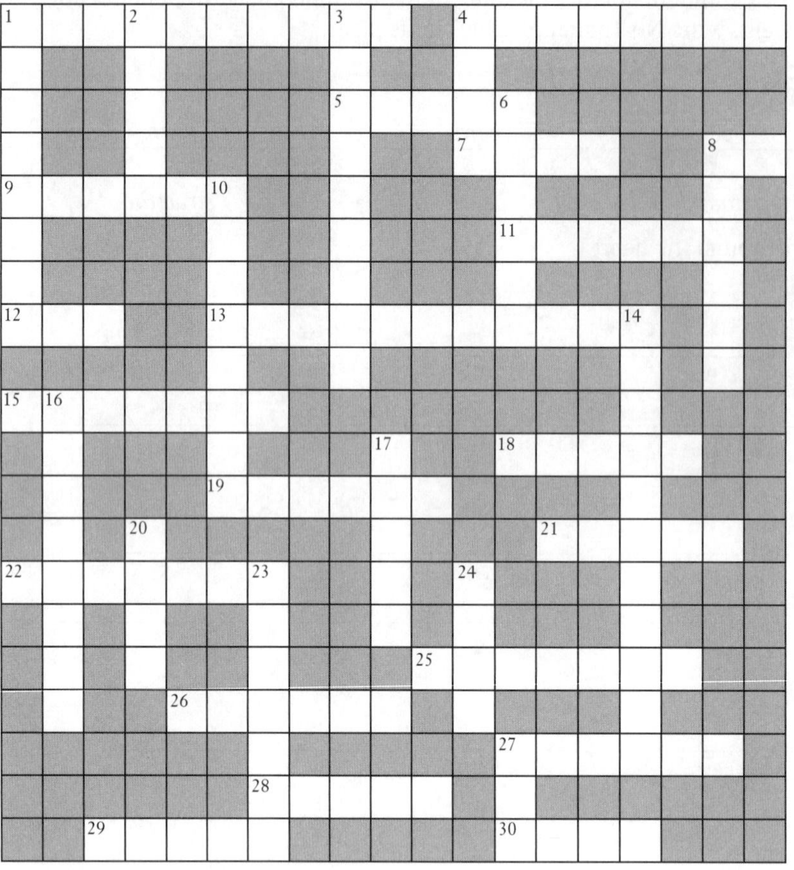

ACROSS

1. Test to determine suitability of mixing donor and recipient blood
4. Containing blood vessels
5. The upper, receiving chambers on each side of the heart
7. Structure described as a mass of differentiated tissue
8. Prothrombin time (abbrev.)
9. Abnormal reduction in the number of RBCs in the circulating blood
11. A coat or layer of tissue, as in a blood vessel
12. Abbreviation for a common hematology test
13. Medical term for red blood cell
15. Medication/therapy for cardiac disease
18. Fluid that circulates within the vascular system
19. Partition that separates the right and left chambers of the heart
21. Muscular organ that receives blood from veins and propels it into arteries
22. Small veins that emerge from capillaries
25. Last-choice AC vein for venipuncture
26. Another name for the bicuspid heart valve
27. Test used to identify the presence of fibrinolysis
28. Fluid derived from excess tissue fluid and similar in composition to plasma
29. Vein structure that helps keep blood flowing toward the heart
30. Soft, insoluble mass found in red-top tube

DOWN

1. Second-choice AC vein for venipuncture
2. Pale-yellow fluid that can be separated from a clotted blood specimen
3. To clot, or change from liquid to solid
4. Blood vessel that returns blood to the heart
6. Pertaining to the large artery arising from the left ventricle
8. Fluid portion of the circulating blood
10. Blood vessels that carry blood away from the heart
14. Term for the thin inner layer of the heart
16. Insufficient blood supply to an area due to obstruction of the blood vessels carrying blood to the area
17. _______coat is composed of WBCs and platelets
20. Colloquial name for the heart, "the ______"
23. Contracting phase of the cardiac cycle
24. Immediately
27. Pathological form of diffuse coagulation (abbrev.)

Chapter Review Questions

1. The thin membrane lining the heart that is continuous with the lining of the blood vessels is the:
   a. endocardium.
   b. epicardium.
   c. myocardium.
   d. pericardium.

2. Partitions that separate the right and left chambers of the heart are called:
   a. chordae tendineae.
   b. cusps.
   c. Purkinje fibers.
   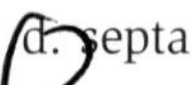
   d. septa.

3. The bicuspid valve in the heart is also called the:
   a. aortic valve.
   b. mitral valve.
   c. pulmonic valve.
   d. tricuspid valve.

4. The function of the right ventricle is to:
   a. deliver blood to the aorta.
   b. deliver blood to the pulmonary artery.
   c. receive blood from the pulmonary vein.
   d. receive blood from the vena cava.

5. A fast heart rate is called:
   a. arrhythmia.
   b. bradycardia.
   c. fibrillations.
   d. tachycardia.

6. The sound of the heartbeat comes from:
   a. contracting myocardium.
   b. firing of the sinoatrial node.
   c. opening and closing of the valves.
   d. resonating interventricular septa.

7. Diastolic blood pressure is the pressure in the arteries during
   a. atrial contraction.
   b. atrial relaxation.
   c. ventricular contraction.
   d. ventricular relaxation.

8. Which of the following arteries carries deoxygenated blood?
   a. Brachial
   b. Femoral
   c. Pulmonary
   d. Radial

9. A vein is defined as a blood vessel that carries
   a. blood away from the heart.
   b. blood to the heart.
   c. deoxygenated blood.
   d. oxygen-rich blood.

10. While selecting a vein for venipuncture, you feel a distinct pulse. What you are feeling is a/an
    a. artery.
    b. nerve.
    c. valve.
    d. vein.

11. A major difference between veins and arteries is that
    a. arteries have a thicker external layer.
    b. arteries have no endothelial layer.
    c. veins have a thicker medial layer.
    d. veins have valves.

12. The outer layer of a blood vessel is called the tunica
    a. adventitia.
    b. interna.
    c. intima.
    d. media.

13. Which of the following veins are most commonly used for venipuncture?
    a. Basilic and median cubital
    b. Cephalic and basilic
    c. Median cubital and cephalic
    d. Radial and basilic

14. Which of the following formed elements is actually part of a bone marrow cell called a megakaryocyte?
    a. Erythrocyte
    b. Granulocyte
    c. Thrombocyte
    d. Reticulocyte

15. Whole blood consists of all of the following except
    a. cells.
    b. fibrin.
    c. plasma.
    d. solutes.

16. A person's blood type is determined by antigens on the surfaces of the
    a. eosinophils.
    b. platelets.
    c. red blood cells.
    d. white blood cells.

17. The third response of the coagulation process is
    a. fibrinolysis.
    b. platelet plug formation.
    c. hemostatic plug formation.
    d. vasoconstriction.

18. When platelets stick to each other during the coagulation process, it is called
    a. aggregation.
    b. adhesion.
    c. infarction.
    d. inhibition.

19. Which of the following is a function of the lymphatic system?
    a. Carry oxygen to the cells
    b. Regulate blood pressure
    c. Remove microorganisms
    d. Synthesize coagulation factors

20. A blood clot circulating in the bloodstream is called a/an
    a. embolism.
    b. embolus.
    c. phlebitis.
    d. thrombus.

CASE STUDIES

Case Study 6-1 Circulatory System Disorders and Diagnostic Tests

A phlebotomist receives a request to collect specimens for stat electrolytes, CK, and AST on a patient with a possible MI. When the phlebotomist arrives to draw the specimen, a physician is with the patient and the patient is explaining that he had been feeling extreme anginal pains for almost an hour now. The physician tells the phlebotomist to go ahead and draw the specimen. The patient has an IV in the left arm near the wrist. There is a sphygmomanometer around the upper right arm.

QUESTIONS

1. What do the abbreviations CK and AST stand for?
2. What circulatory system structure is being evaluated by the ordered tests?
3. Tell what the abbreviation MI stands for and explain what it means in nonmedical terms.
4. What does angina have to do with the patient's possible diagnosis of MI?
5. What is a sphygmomanometer, and can the phlebotomist use that arm to draw blood?

Case Study 6-2 Circulatory System Disorders, Diagnostic Tests, and Vein Selection

A phlebotomist receives a request to collect a specimen for a PT and D-dimer on a patient. The phlebotomist remembers drawing the patient in the ER when he was complaining of leg pain. Because the patient was a difficult draw, the phlebotomist wanted to draw from an ankle vein, but the physician would not give permission. The patient was subsequently diagnosed with DVT. When the phlebotomist received the next request on this patient, he still couldn't find a good vein in the AC area, but he noticed that the patient had a large vein on the underside of the wrist. Before he could collect from the wrist area, he was called to a stat in ER.

QUESTIONS

1. Should the phlebotomist draw from the vein on the underside of the wrist? Why or why not?
2. What do PT and DVT stand for?
3. What body process is being evaluated by the requested tests?
4. What type of specimen is required: serum, plasma or whole blood?
5. Give a reason for your selection of specimen type.

(6-1)

1. CREATINE KINASE, ASPARTATE AMINOTRASFERASE,
2. THE HEART
3. MYCARDIAL INFARCIAN
4. CHEST PAIN / HEART ATTACK
5. NO, ITS A BLOOD PRESSURE CUFF

(6-2)

1. NO, BECAUSE IT IS A DELICATE/COMPACT AREA AND THERES SO MANY NERVES.
2. PT IS PROTHROMBIN TIME AND DVT IS DEEP VENUS THROMBOSIS OR BLOOD CLOT.
3. VASCULAR
4. PLASMA
5.

UNIT II CROSSWORD EXERCISE

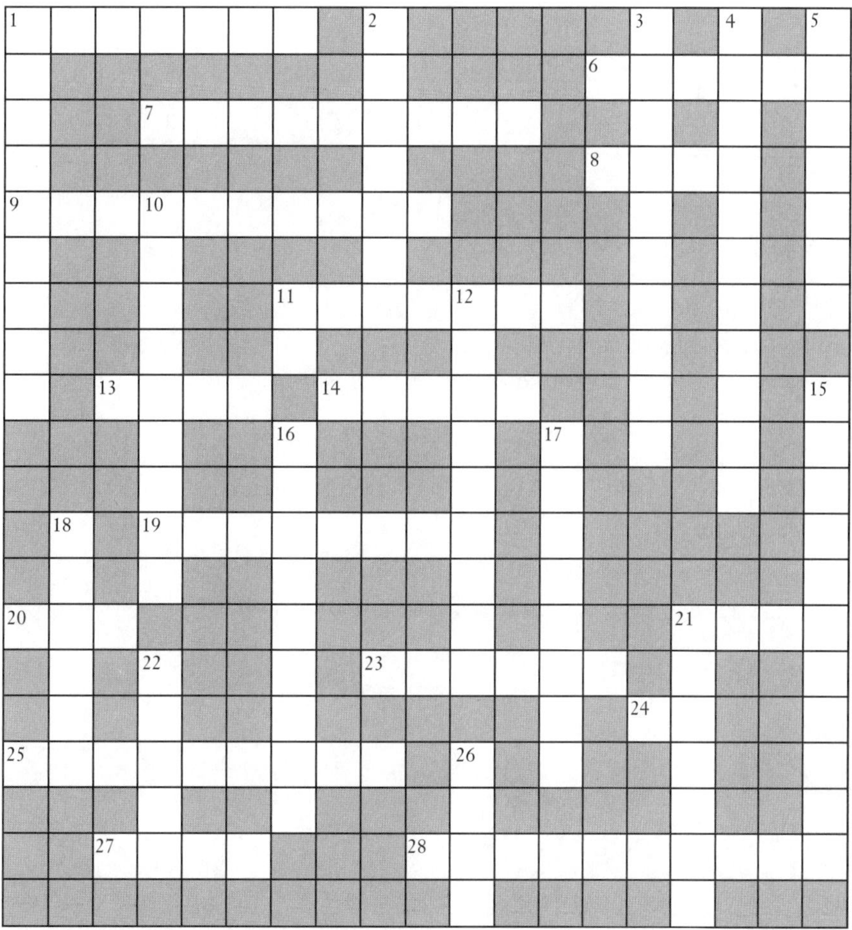

ACROSS

1. Tiny sacs in the lungs where oxygen exchange takes place
6. Fundamental working unit of the nervous system
7. Sometimes called the master gland
8. Veins in this area are not allowed to be punctured without physician's permission
9. Breakdown of complex substances into simple ones
11. Last-choice AC vein for venipuncture
13. A mass of lymphatic tissue through which lymph flows
14. Normally clear pale-yellow fluid that can be separated from a clotted specimen
19. Circulation pathway that carries oxygenated blood throughout the body
20. Blood group system
21. Partial thromboplastin time (pl. abbrev.)
23. Word element that precedes a word root
24. Prothrombin time (abbrev.)
25. Type of gland that secretes directly into the bloodstream
27. Vessel that typically carries deoxygenated blood
28. Blood coagulation is a component of this process

DOWN

1. Without blood or lymph vessels
2. A type of cell duplication that involves doubling of DNA and cell division
3. Iron-containing pigment that gives RBCs their color
4. Red blood cell
5. The science of the structural composition of living things
10. Body process in which simple compounds are converted into complex substances
11. Test that checks platelet function (abbrev.)
12. White blood cell
15. State of equilibrium of the internal environment of the body
16. Coagulation pathway activated by tissue thromboplastin
17. Viscid fluid found in the joints
18. Protein filament formed by action of thrombin on fibrinogen
21. Coagulation cascade involves an intrinsic and extrinsic _____
22. Lying face down
26. One of the waste products of metabolism

UNIT III BLOOD COLLECTION PROCEDURES

CHAPTER 7

Blood Collection Equipment, Additives, and Order of Draw

OBJECTIVES

Study the information in your textbook that corresponds to each objective to prepare yourself for the activities in this chapter.

1. Define the key terms and abbreviations listed at the beginning of this chapter.
2. List, describe, and explain the purpose of the equipment and supplies needed to collect blood by venipuncture.
3. Compare and contrast antiseptics and disinfectants and give examples of each.
4. Identify appropriate phlebotomy needles by length, gauge, and any associated color coding.
5. List and describe evacuated tube system (ETS) and syringe system components, explain how each system works, and tell how to determine which system and components to use.
6. Identify the general categories of additives used in blood collection, list the various additives within each category, and describe how each additive works.
7. Describe the color coding used to identify the presence or absence of additives in blood collection tubes and name the additive, laboratory departments, and individual tests associated with the various color-coded tubes.
8. List the "order of draw" when multiple tubes are being collected and explain why it is important.

Matching

Use choices only once unless otherwise indicated.

MATCHING 7-1: KEY TERMS AND DESCRIPTIONS

Match each key term with the *best* description.

Key Terms (1–16)

1. _____ ACD
2. _____ Additive
3. _____ Anticoagulant
4. _____ Antiglycolytic agent
5. _____ Antiseptics
6. _____ Bevel
7. _____ Butterfly needle
8. _____ Clot activator
9. _____ Disinfectant
10. _____ EDTA
11. _____ ETS
12. _____ Evacuated tube
13. _____ Gauge
14. _____ Glycolysis
15. _____ Heparin
16. _____ Hub

Descriptions (1–16)

A. Abbreviation for the collection system typically used for routine venipuncture
B. Additive that prevents the breakdown of glucose by the cells
C. Additive used for immunohematology tests such as DNA and HLA typing
D. Anticoagulant that inhibits the formation of thrombin
E. Anticoagulant that preserves cell shape and structure and inhibits platelet clumping
F. Breakdown or metabolism of glucose by blood cells
G. Coagulation-enhancing substance, such as silica
H. End of the needle that attaches to the blood collection device
I. Number that is related to the diameter of the needle lumen
J. Point of a needle that is cut on a slant for ease of skin entry
K. Premeasured vacuum tube that is color-coded based on its additive
L. Solutions used to kill microorganisms on surfaces and instruments
M. Substance added to a blood collection tube
N. Substance that prevents blood from clotting
O. Substances used for skin cleaning that inhibit the growth of bacteria
P. Winged infusion blood collection set

Key Terms (17–31)

17. _____ Hypodermic needle
18. _____ Lumen
19. _____ Multisample needle
20. _____ Order of draw
21. _____ Potassium oxalate
22. _____ PST
23. _____ Shaft
24. _____ Sharps container
25. _____ Silica
26. _____ Sodium citrate
27. _____ Sodium fluoride
28. _____ SPS
29. _____ SST
30. _____ Thixotropic gel
31. _____ Winged infusion set

Descriptions (17–31)

A. Additive used in blood culture collection
B. Anticoagulant commonly used to preserve coagulation factors
C. Anticoagulant commonly used with an antiglycolytic agent
D. Butterfly needle
E. Clot activator
F. Gel tube for separation of cells and serum
G. Heparinized gel tube for separation of cells and plasma
H. Internal space of a vessel or tube
I. Long cylindrical portion of a needle
J. Most common antiglycolytic agent
K. Special puncture-resistant leakproof disposable container
L. Special sequence in which tubes are filled during a multiple-tube draw
M. Synthetic substance used to separate cells from serum or plasma
N. Type of needle used to collect several tubes during a single venipuncture
O. Type of needle used when collecting blood with a syringe

MATCHING 7–2: MATCH THE ADDITIVE WITH ITS PRIMARY FUNCTION

Choices may be used more than once.

Additive

1. ______ ACD
2. ______ CPD
3. ______ EDTA
4. ______ Heparin
5. ______ Potassium oxalate
6. ______ Silica
7. ______ Sodium citrate
8. ______ Sodium fluoride
9. ______ SPS
10. ______ Thixotropic gel

Primary Function

A. Anticoagulant
B. Antiglycolytic agent
C. Clot activator
D. Serum/plasma separator

MATCHING 7–3: MATCH THE ADDITIVE WITH THE TYPE OF ACTION

Choices may be used more than once.

Additive

1. ______ Citrate
2. ______ EDTA
3. ______ Heparin
4. ______ Potassium oxalate
5. ______ Silica
6. ______ Sodium fluoride
7. ______ Thixotropic gel

Type of Action

A. Binds calcium
B. Enhances coagulation
C. Inhibits thrombin
D. Physical barrier
E. Preserves glucose

Labeling Exercises

LABELING EXERCISE 7-1: TUBE STOPPER COLORS AND ADDITIVES

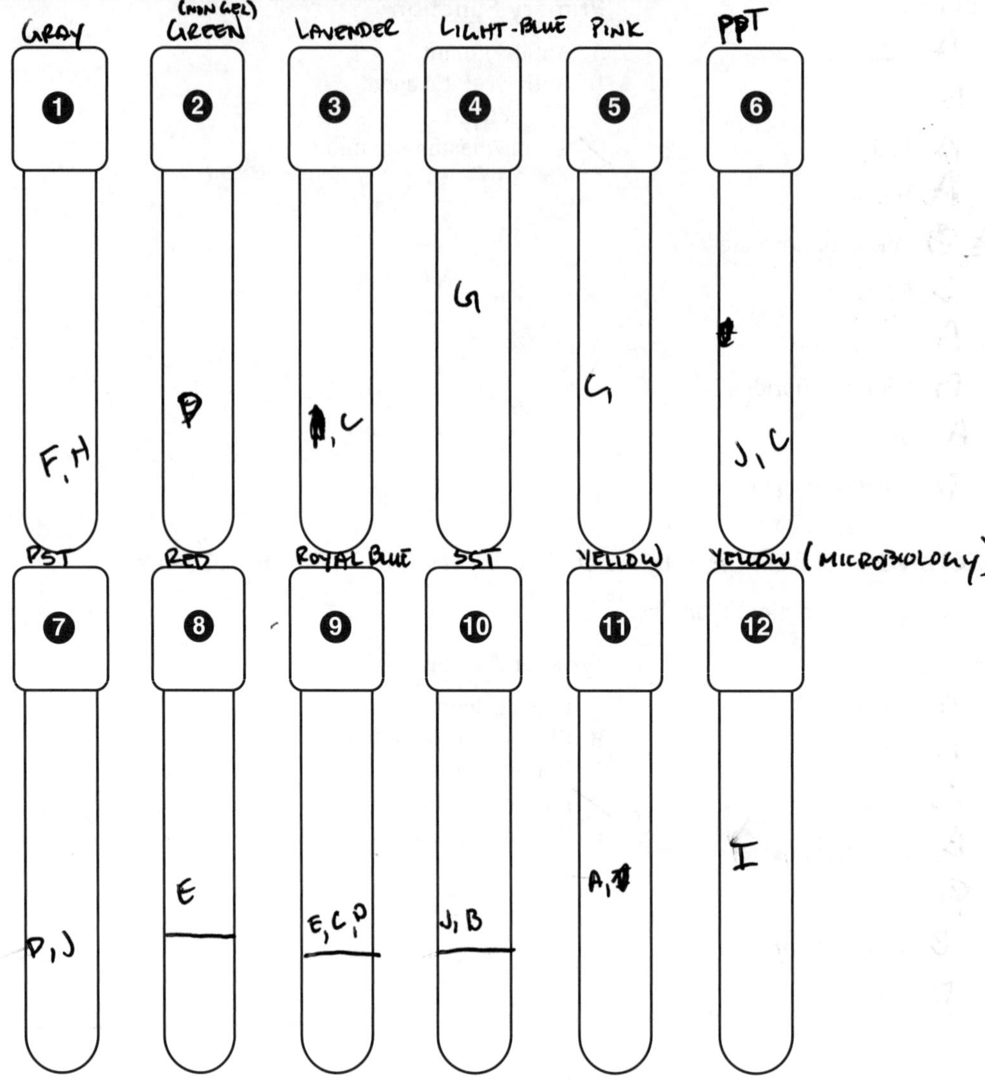

Color the tube stoppers of the following ETS plastic tubes according to the list of tubes below. If the tube contains gel, color the area of the tube that would contain the gel yellow. Using the list of additives, write the letter(s) of the possible tube additive(s) inside the corresponding tube. *Note*: Additive choices may be used more than once, and some tube choices may have more than one additive.

Tubes

1. Gray top
2. Green top (nongel)
3. Lavender top
4. Light-blue top
5. Pink top
6. PPT
7. PST
8. Red top
9. Royal-blue top
10. SST
11. Yellow top (blood bank)
12. Yellow top (microbiology)

Additives

a. Acid citrate dextrose (ACD)
b. Clot activator (silica)
c. EDTA
d. Heparin
e. No additive
f. Potassium oxalate
g. Sodium citrate
h. Sodium fluoride
i. Sodium polyanethol sulfonate (SPS)
j. Thixotropic gel

LABELING EXERCISE 7-2: TUBE STOPPER COLORS AND ORDER OF DRAW

Identify the stopper color of the tube required for the following types of tests assuming that they would all be collected from the same patient at the same time. Then, in the order of draw from left to right, color the stoppers of the following tubes to correspond to the tubes required for the types of tests.

Tube Stopper Color	Type of Test
1. GRAY	Chemistry test (antiglycolytic agent required)
2. GREEN	Chemistry test (plasma required)
3. SST	Chemistry test (serum required)
4. LAVENDER / PINK	Coagulation test
5. LIGHT BLUE	Hematology test

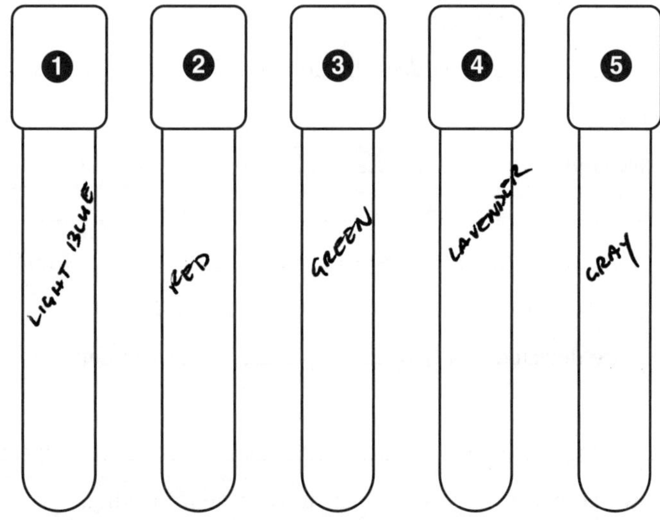

Knowledge Drills

KNOWLEDGE DRILL 7-1: CAUTION AND KEY POINT RECOGNITION

The following sentences are taken from Caution and Key Point statements found throughout the text of Chapter 7. Using the TEXTBOOK, fill in the blanks with the missing information.

1. According to (A) ____________ regulations, if the (B) ____________ does not have a (C) ____________ feature, the equipment it is used with (such as tube holder or syringe) must have a (D) ____________ feature to minimize the chance of an accidental needlestick.
2. Always check the (A) ____________ ____________ on a tube before using it, and never use a tube that has (B) ____________ or has been (C) ____________.
3. An underfilled (A) ____________ tube will have an incorrect blood-to-additive (B) ____________, which can cause (D) ____________ test results.
4. Cleaning with an (A) ____________ reduces the number of (B) ____________ but does not (C) ____________ the site.
5. (A) ____________ of hands after (B) ____________ removal is essential.
6. Heparinized (A) ____________ is preferred over (B) ____________ for (C) ____________ tests because when blood clots, (D) ____________ is released from (E) ____________ into the serum and can falsely elevate results.
7. If (A) ____________ are detected in a (B) ____________ specimen, it cannot be used for testing and must be (C) ____________.
8. *Never* (A) ____________ or otherwise (B) ____________ ____________ a specimen, as this can cause (C) ____________, which makes most specimens unsuitable for testing.
9. *Never* transfer blood collected in an (A) ____________ tube into another (B) ____________ tube, even if the (C) ____________ are the same.
10. (A) ____________ regulations require that the tube holder with (B) ____________ ____________ be disposed of as a (C) ____________ after use and never be removed from the (D) ____________ and reused.
11. The (A) ____________ tube collected with a (B) ____________ will underfill because of the (C) ____________ in the tubing. If the tube contains an (D) ____________, the blood-to-additive ratio will be affected.
12. The (A) ____________ ratio of blood to (B) ____________ in light-blue (C) ____________ ____________ tubes is (D) ____________; therefore, it is extremely important to fill them to the stated capacity.

KNOWLEDGE DRILL 7-2: SCRAMBLED WORDS

Unscramble the following words using the hints given in parenthesis. Write the correct spelling of the scrambled word on the line next to it.

1. cavmuu VACUUM (negative pressure)
2. clabeh BLEACH (sodium hypochlorite)
3. eggua GAUGE (measure of diameter)
4. mulen LUMEN (the space within)
5. pheanri HEPARIN (it inhibits thrombin)
6. poxihirctot THIXOTOPIC (type of gel)
7. quinretout TOURNQUIT (used to restrict blood flow)
8. reatict CITRATE (coagulation tube additive)
9. treyfblut BUTTERFLY (winged infusion set)
10. veldrean LAVENDER (EDTA tube stopper color)
11. voyarcrer CARRYOVER (transfer from one tube to another)
12. zitsieran SANITIZER (used to decontaminate hands)

KNOWLEDGE DRILL 7-3: STOPPER COLORS, ADDITIVES, AND DEPARTMENTS

Fill in the blanks of the following table with the missing information.

Stopper Color(s)	Additive	Department(s)
Light blue	Sodium citrate	(1) ____________
Red	(2) ____________	Chemistry, Blood Bank, Serology/Immunology
Red	Clot activator	(3) ____________
Red/light gray Clear	(4) ____________	NA (discard purpose only)
Red/black (tiger) Red/gold (5) ____________	Clot activator and (6) ____________	Chemistry
Green/gray (7) ____________	Lithium heparin and gel separator	Chemistry
Green	Lithium heparin Sodium heparin Aluminum heparin	(8) ____________
Lavender (purple)	EDTA	(9) ____________
(10) ____________	EDTA	Blood bank
Gray	Sodium fluoride and (11) ____________ Sodium fluoride and (12) ____________ Sodium fluoride	Chemistry
Orange Gray/yellow	(13) ____________	Chemistry
Royal blue	(14) ____________ (15) ____________ Sodium (16) ____________	Chemistry
Tan (plastic)	(17) ____________	Chemistry
Yellow	(18) ____________ ____________ (SPS)	Microbiology
Yellow	Acid citrate dextrose (19) (____________)	(20) ____________ / Immunohematology

Skills Drills

SKILLS DRILL 7-1: REQUISITION ACTIVITY

Identify the tests ordered on the following requisition. List the tests below in the order of draw and identify the stopper color and additive of the tubes that will most likely be collected for the tests indicated.

Order of Draw	Tube Stopper Color and Additive
1. PT - (PROTIME)	LIGHT BLUE (Na CITRATE)
2. TYPE + SCREEN (SERUM SPECIMEN)	RED (NONE)
3. H + H	LAVENDER (POTASSIUM, EDTA)
4. LYTES (ELECTROLYTES)	~~GRAY (K-OXALATE, Na FLUORIDE)~~ GREEN (GENERAL CHEMISTRY) HEPARIN

Any Hospital USA
1123 West Physician Drive
Any Town USA

Laboratory Test Requisition

PATIENT INFORMATION:

Name: Doe (last) John (first) T (MI)

Identification Number: 036152912 Birth Date: 12/07/43

Referring Physician: Smarte, John

Date to be Collected: 06/28/2011 Time to be Collected: ____

Special Instructions: **STAT**

TEST(S) ORDERED:

	Chemistry		**Coagulation**	
	NH4 (Ammonia)		D-dimer	
	Bili (Bilirubin, total & direct)	√	PT (protime)	LIGHT BLUE
	BMP (basic metabolic panel)		PTT (partial thromboplastin time)	
	BUN (Blood urea nitrogen)		**Hematology**	
	Chol (cholesterol)		CBC (complete blood count)	
	EtOH (alcohol)		ESR (erythrocyte sed rate)	
	Gluc (glucose)		Hgb (hemoglobin)	
~~GRAY~~ GREEN √	Lytes (electrolytes)	√	H & H (hemoglobin & Hematocrit)	LAVENDER
	Lact (lactic acid/lactate)		RBC (Red blood cell count)	
	PSA (prostatic specific antigen)		WBC (White blood cell count)	
Other	√	*Type & Screen (serum specimen requested)*		RED

SKILLS DRILL 7-2: WORD BUILDING

Divide each word into all of its elements (parts); prefix (P), word root (WR), combining vowel (CV), and suffix (S). Write the word part, its definition, and the meaning of the word on the corresponding lines. If the word does not have a particular element, write NA (not applicable) in its place.

Example: Antiglycolytic

Elements *anti* / *glyc* / *o* / *lytic*
P WR CV S

Definitions *against* / *sugar* / ____ / *pertaining to breakdown*

Meaning: Against the breakdown of sugar (glucose)

1. Hypodermic

Elements ________ / ________ / ____ / ________
P WR CV S

Definitions ________ / ________ / ____ / ________

Meaning:

2. Dermatitis

Elements ________ / ________ / ____ / ________
P WR CV S

Definitions ________ / ________ / ____ / ________

Meaning:

3. Antiseptic

Elements ________ / ________ / ____ / ________
P WR CV S

Definitions ________ / ________ / ____ / ________

Meaning:

4. Microorganism

Elements ________ / ________ / ____ / ________
P WR CV S

Definitions ________ / ________ / ____ / ________

Meaning:

5. Vascular

Elements ________ / ________ / ____ / ________
P WR CV S

Definitions ________ / ________ / ____ / ________

Meaning:

6. Intradermal

Elements ________ / ________ / ____ / ________
P WR CV S

Definitions ________ / ________ / ____ / ________

Meaning:

Crossword

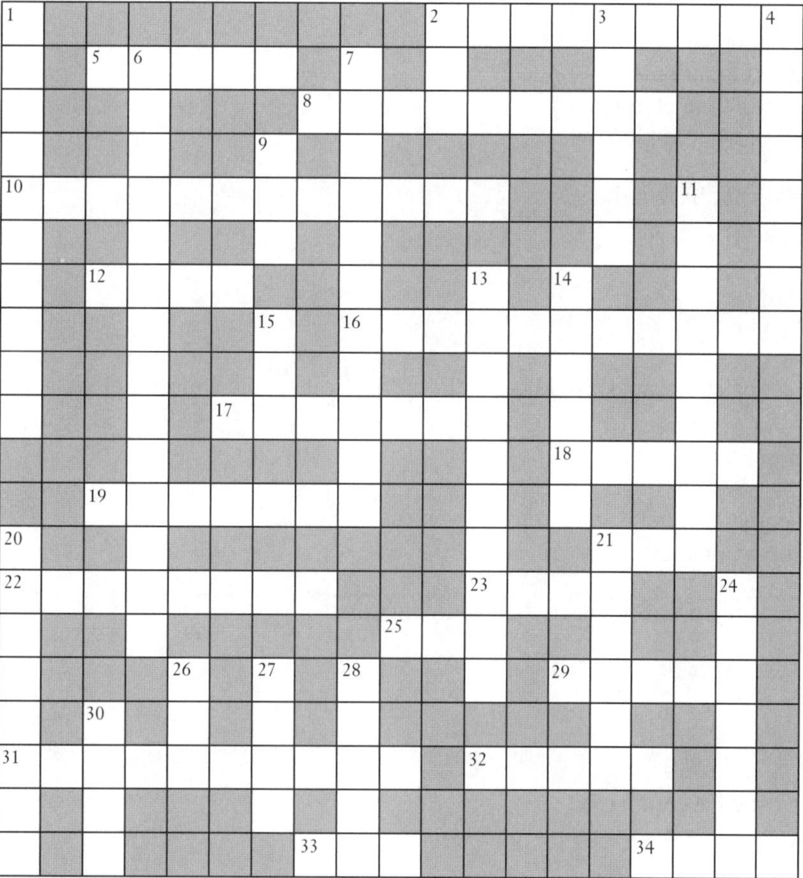

ACROSS

2. EDTA or oxalate anticoagulants are usually salts of this element
5. Diameter of the lumen of the needle
8. Winged infusion set
10. Solution used to remove or kill microbes
12. It forms in a tube of blood that does not have anticoagulant in it
16. Used to clean the site before puncture (plural)
17. Another name for cap on evacuated tubes
18. Internal space of a tube or blood vessel
19. Used to obtain blood when veins are very fragile
21. Gold top tube that contains separator gel (abbrev.)
22. Any substance added to an evacuated collection tube
23. Agency that mandates and enforces safe working conditions
25. The time it takes to turn around test results
29. End of the needle that is cut on a slant for ease of insertion
31. Inflammation of the skin
32. Type of examination glove
33. Only clot activator is found in this plastic evacuated tube
34. Phlebotomy standards are set by this institute

DOWN

1. Name for a sterile syringe needle
2. Heparin gel barrier tube (abbrev.)
3. Clot activator in SST
4. Short for microorganisms
6. Literally means "against glucose breakdown"
7. Type of needle used with an ETS
9. Barrier used in separator tubes, thixotropic _______
11. Items needed for phlebotomy procedure
13. Tiny clots invisible to the eye
14. 21-gauge or 22-gauge _______
15. EDTA gel barrier tube abbrev.
20. ETS cap color that indicates EDTA
21. This device must be activated before a needle is discarded
24. ETS part that contains the tube during venipuncture (plural)
26. Agency that regulates food and drugs (abbrev.)
27. Name of a vessel that returns blood to the heart
28. Object on which a blood smear is made
30. Tube used to collect blood alcohol

Chapter Review Questions

1. An antiglycolytic agent:
   a. enhances coagulation.
   b. inhibits thrombin formation.
   c. keeps the specimen from clotting.
   d. prevents the breakdown of glucose.

2. Sharps containers do not have to be:
   a. marked "biohazard."
   b. disposable.
   c. puncture-resistant.
   d. recyclable.

3. Which of the following substances would be the best thing to use to disinfect a blood spill on a lab countertop prior to cleanup?
   a. A 1:10 dilution of bleach
   b. 70% Isopropyl alcohol
   c. Antibacterial soap and water
   d. Povidone–iodine swab sticks

4. This needle is the standard needle for routine venipuncture.
   a. 20 gauge
   b. 21 gauge
   c. 22 gauge
   d. 23 gauge

5. Needles are color-coded according to:
   a. expiration date.
   b. gauge.
   c. length.
   d. manufacturer.

6. The most common, direct, and efficient means of venipuncture is:
   a. butterfly and tube holder.
   b. butterfly and syringe.
   c. ETS needle and tube holder.
   d. needle and syringe.

7. Which of the following would be the best choice of equipment for drawing a small hand vein?
   a. A 21-gauge needle and syringe
   b. A 22-gauge needle and ETS holder
   c. A 23-gauge butterfly and ETS holder
   d. A 25-gauge butterfly needle and syringe

8. Which of the following equipment is required in collecting blood by syringe?
   a. Multisample needle
   b. Tube holder
   c. Transfer device
   d. Winged infusion set

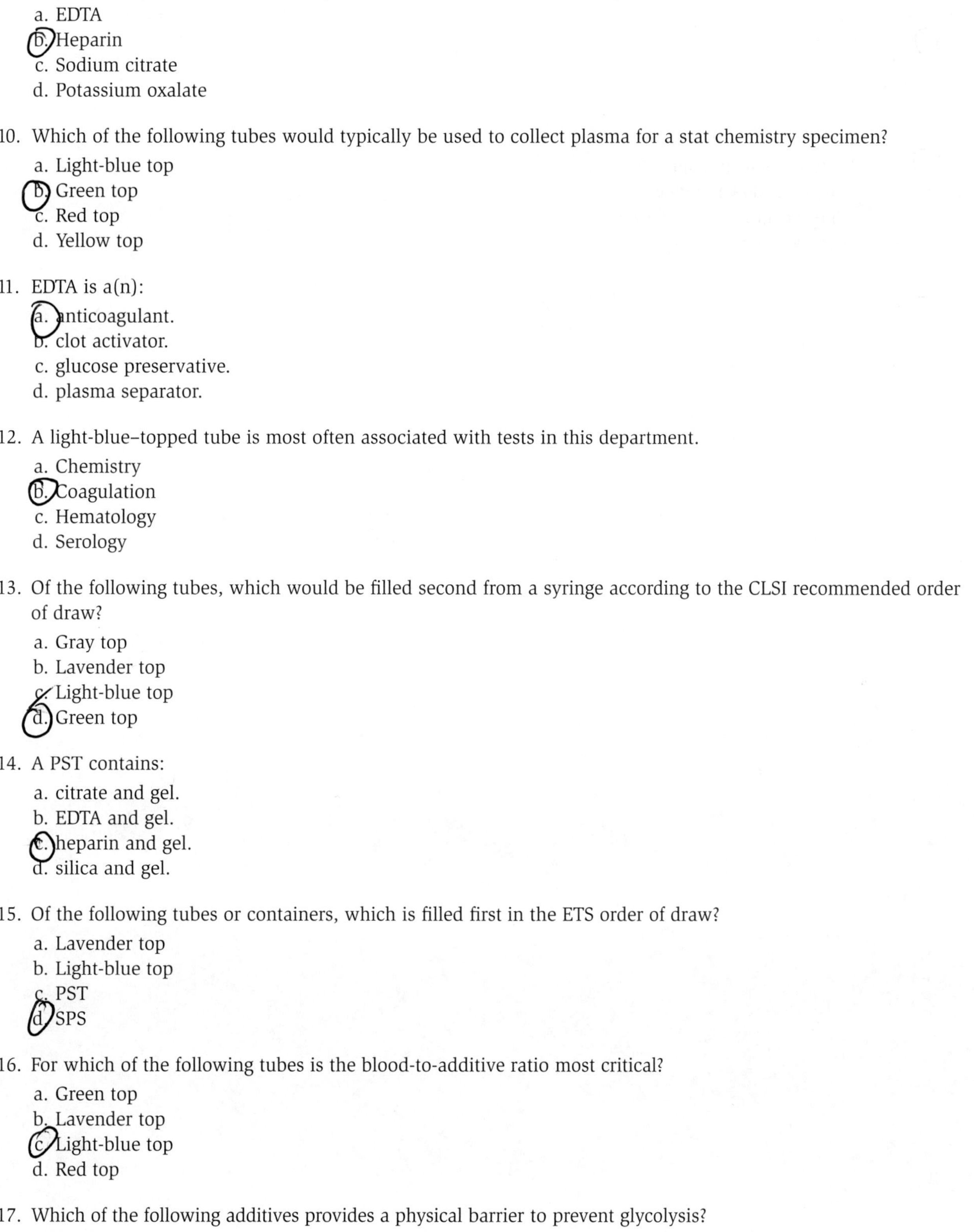

9. Which anticoagulant prevents coagulation by inhibiting thrombin formation?
   a. EDTA
   b. Heparin
   c. Sodium citrate
   d. Potassium oxalate

10. Which of the following tubes would typically be used to collect plasma for a stat chemistry specimen?
    a. Light-blue top
    b. Green top
    c. Red top
    d. Yellow top

11. EDTA is a(n):
    a. anticoagulant.
    b. clot activator.
    c. glucose preservative.
    d. plasma separator.

12. A light-blue–topped tube is most often associated with tests in this department.
    a. Chemistry
    b. Coagulation
    c. Hematology
    d. Serology

13. Of the following tubes, which would be filled second from a syringe according to the CLSI recommended order of draw?
    a. Gray top
    b. Lavender top
    c. Light-blue top
    d. Green top

14. A PST contains:
    a. citrate and gel.
    b. EDTA and gel.
    c. heparin and gel.
    d. silica and gel.

15. Of the following tubes or containers, which is filled first in the ETS order of draw?
    a. Lavender top
    b. Light-blue top
    c. PST
    d. SPS

16. For which of the following tubes is the blood-to-additive ratio most critical?
    a. Green top
    b. Lavender top
    c. Light-blue top
    d. Red top

17. Which of the following additives provides a physical barrier to prevent glycolysis?
    a. EDTA
    b. Silica
    c. Sodium fluoride
    d. Thixotropic gel

18. Which of the following tubes contains an anticoagulant that works by binding calcium?
    a. Green top
    b. Light-blue top
    c. PST
    d. SST

19. What is the purpose of a royal blue–topped tube?
    a. Minimize trace-element contamination
    b. Prevent the breakdown of glucose
    c. Prevent the specimen from clotting
    d. Protect the specimen from light

CASE STUDIES

Case Study 7-1 Butterfly Use and Order of Draw

Maria, who was recently hired in her first job as a phlebotomist, has been sent to the ICU to collect a stat hemoglobin and hematocrit (H&H) and protime on a patient. The patient is an elderly woman whose left arm has an intravenous (IV) line. Maria checks the right arm and finds a small but suitable vein. She decides to use a butterfly with the evacuated tube system and selects the following tubes from her blood collection equipment carrier: a light blue top for the protime, which is a coagulation test, and a lavender top for the H&H, which is a hematology test. The patient's nurse asks Maria how long she thinks it will take because she wants to give the patient a shot in that arm. Maria tells her that she has only two tubes to collect so it shouldn't take long. The nurse leaves. Maria makes a successful venipuncture, fills the light blue–topped tube and mixes it gently by inverting it four times. Then she fills the lavender-top tube. After finishing the draw, properly labeling the tubes, and checking and bandaging her patient, she returns to the lab. Specimen processing immediately rejects the protime and asks her to re-collect it.

QUESTIONS

1. Why do you think specimen processing rejected the protime?
2. How did the way Maria collected the specimen cause the problem?
3. Why does the lab reject tubes with this problem?
4. What can Maria do differently when she re-collects the specimen?

Case Study 7-2 Syringe Use and Order of Draw

A phlebotomist named Jeff has a request to collect a CBC on a postop patient. He has drawn the patient before and is aware that the patient is a "difficult" draw. He elects to use a 5-mL syringe and a 22-gauge needle on a small cephalic vein on the patient's right arm. The venipuncture is successful, and Jeff is in the middle of filling the syringe when the patient's nurse enters the room and tells him that the patient's physician wants to add electrolytes to the request. Jeff tells her that it is not a problem; he will collect a green-top tube also. He finishes the draw, attaches a transfer device, and quickly grabs the smallest tubes he can find, a 3-mL green top for the electrolytes and a 3-mL lavender top for the CBC. He puts 2 mL of blood into the green top and then 3 mL into the lavender top. He labels the tubes and writes "difficult draw" on the green top. Later a chemistry technician tells him that the patient's sodium results are off the wall and contamination is suspected. He is asked to redraw the specimen.

QUESTIONS

1. Could the problem have to do with the order of draw? Why or why not?
2. What else could have caused the problem?
3. Technically, there is another problem with the green top Jeff collected. What is it?

CHAPTER

8

Venipuncture Specimen Collection Procedures

OBJECTIVES

Study the information in your textbook that corresponds to each objective to prepare yourself for the activities in this chapter.

1. Define the key terms and abbreviations listed at the beginning of the chapter.
2. Describe the test request process, identify the types of requisitions used, and list required requisition information.
3. List and define test status designations, identify status priorities, and describe the procedure to follow for each status designation.
4. Describe proper "bedside manner" and how to handle special situations associated with patient contact.
5. Explain the importance of proper patient identification and describe what information is verified, how to handle discrepancies, and what to do if a patient's ID band is missing.
6. Describe how to prepare patients for testing, how to answer inquiries concerning tests, and what to do if a patient objects to a test.
7. Describe how to verify fasting and other diet requirements and what to do when diet requirements have not been met.
8. Describe each step in the venipuncture procedure, list necessary information found on specimen tube labels, and list the acceptable reasons for inability to collect a specimen.
9. Describe collection procedures when using a butterfly or syringe and the proper way to safely dispense blood into tubes following syringe collection.
10. Describe unique requirements associated with drawing blood from special populations including pediatric, geriatric, and long-term care patients.

Matching

Use each choice only once unless otherwise indicated.

MATCHING 8-1: KEY TERMS AND DESCRIPTIONS

Match each key term with the *best* description.

Key Terms (1–12)

1. ______ Accession
2. ______ Anchor
3. ______ Arm/wrist band
4. ______ ASAP
5. ______ Barcode
6. ______ Bedside manner
7. ______ Concentric circles
8. ______ DNR/DNAR
9. ______ EMLA
10. ______ Fasting
11. ______ Hospice
12. ______ ID band/bracelet

Descriptions (1–12)

A. A eutectic mixture of local anesthetics
B. As soon as possible
C. Behavior of a healthcare provider toward a patient or as perceived by a patient
D. Do not resuscitate/do not attempt resuscitation
E. Identification bracelet (abbrev.)
F. No food or drink except water for 8 to 12 hours
G. Record in the order received
H. Secure firmly, as in holding a vein in place by pulling the skin taut with the thumb
I. Series of black stripes and white spaces that correspond to letters and numbers
J. Starting from the center and moving outward in ever-widening circles
K. Two other names for an identification band/bracelet
L. Type of care for terminally ill patients

Key Terms (13–24)

13. ______ ID card
14. ______ MR number
15. ______ Needle phobia
16. ______ Needle sheath
17. ______ NPO
18. ______ Palpate
19. ______ Patency
20. ______ Patient ID
21. ______ Preop/postop
22. ______ Reflux
23. ______ Requisition
24. ______ Stat

Descriptions (13–24)

A. Backflow of blood from the tube into the vein during a draw
B. Before an operation or surgery/after an operation or surgery
C. Clinic-issued patient identification document
D. Covering or cap of a needle
E. Form on which test orders are entered and sent to the lab
F. Immediately (from the Latin *statim,* meaning "immediately")
G. Intense fear of needles
H. Medical record number used for patient ID
I. Nothing by mouth (from Latin *nil per os*)
J. Process of verifying a patient's identity
K. State of being freely open
L. To examine by feel or touch

MATCHING 8-2: SITUATION AND ACTION

Match the following venipuncture procedure situations with an acceptable action to take.

Situation

1. _____ Conflicting permission statement
2. _____ ID band not on the patient's arm
3. _____ Needle-phobic patient
4. _____ Outpatient is chewing gum
5. _____ Patient asks for the purpose of the test
6. _____ Patient initially objects to testing
7. _____ Specimen must be fasting but patient has eaten
8. _____ Unconscious patient
9. _____ You are a phlebotomy student
10. _____ You need to verify patient ID

Action

A. Actively involve the patient in this procedure.
B. Advise the patient to ask the nurse or physician.
C. Ask someone to help steady the patient's arm.
D. Ask the patient to remove it.
E. Check the ankle after asking the patient's permission.
F. Consult with the nurse or physician before proceeding.
G. Do not draw blood without the patient's consent.
H. Have the most skilled phlebotomist draw the specimen.
I. Make certain that the patient knows this information.
J. Remind the patient that the doctor needs the test results.

MATCHING 8-3: GERIATRIC PATIENT TESTS AND INDICATIONS-FOR ORDERING

Match the test commonly ordered on geriatric patients (text Table 8-2) to the typical indication for ordering.

Test

1. _____ ANA/RNA/RF
2. _____ CBC
3. _____ BUN/creatinine
4. _____ Calcium/magnesium
5. _____ Electrolytes
6. _____ ESR
7. _____ Glucose
8. _____ PT/PTT
9. _____ SPEP, IPEP
10. _____ VDRL/FTA

Typical Indication for Ordering

A. Detect and monitor diabetes. Abnormal levels can cause confusion, seizures, or coma or lead to peripheral neuropathy.
B. Detect inflammation; identify collagen vascular diseases.
C. Determine hemoglobin levels, detect infection, and identify blood disorders.
D. Determine sodium and potassium levels critical to proper nervous system function.
E. Diagnose kidney function disorders that may be responsible for problems such as confusion, coma, seizures, and tremors.
F. Diagnose lupus and rheumatoid arthritis, which can affect nervous system function.
G. Identify abnormal levels associated with seizures and muscle problems.
H. Identify protein or immune globulin disorders that can lead to nerve damage.
I. Monitor blood-thinning medications; important in heart conditions, coagulation problems, and stroke management.
J. Diagnose or rule out syphilis, which can cause nerve damage and dementia.

Labeling Exercises

LABELING EXERCISE 8-1: PATIENT ID AND BLOOD SPECIMEN LABEL

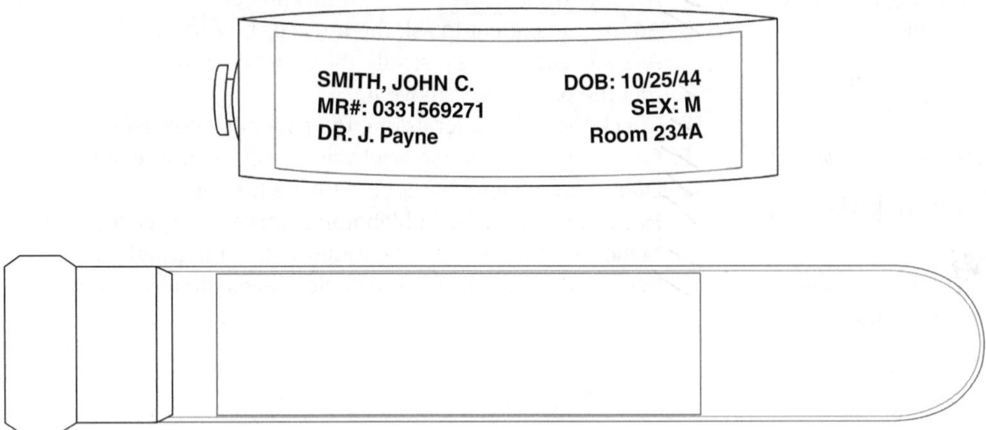

You correctly identified and collected a CBC specimen on May 03, 2011, at 0815 hours from an inpatient who was wearing the ID band shown. Fill out the specimen label on the above tube for this patient. Color the tube stopper the correct color for the test that was collected.

LABELING EXERCISE 8-2: REQUISITION AND BLOOD SPECIMEN LABEL

Any Hospital USA
1123 West Physician Drive
Any Town USA

Laboratory Test Requisition

PATIENT INFORMATION:

Name: Doe (last) Jane (first) A (MI)

Identification Number: 0331724395 Birth Date: 06/14/65

Referring Physician: Coleman

Date to be Collected: 05/04/2011 Time to be Collected: 0600

Special Instructions: NA

TEST(S) REQUIRED:

____ NH4 – Ammonia	____ Gluc – glucose
____ Bili – Bilirubin, total & direct	____ Hgb – hemoglobin
____ BMP – basic metabolic panel	____ Lact – lactic acid/lactate
____ BUN - Blood urea nitrogen	____ Plt. Ct. – platelet count
____ Lytes – electrolytes	X PT – prothrombin time
____ CBC – complete blood count	____ PTT – partial thromboplastin time
____ Chol – cholesterol	____ RPR – rapid plasma reagin
____ ESR – erythrocyte sed rate	____ T&S – type and screen
____ EtOH - alcohol	____ PSA – prostate specific antigen
____ D-dimer	Other ____________

You correctly identified and collected a blood specimen from an inpatient at 0600 hours using the following requisition. Fill out the label shown on the above tube for this patient. Color the tube stopper the correct color for the test that was collected.

Knowledge Drills

KNOWLEDGE DRILL 8-1: CAUTION AND KEY POINT RECOGNITION

The following sentences are taken from Caution or Key Point statements found throughout the Chapter 8 text. Using the TEXTBOOK, fill in the blanks with the missing information.

1. *Never* verify information from an ID band that is not (A) ____________ to the (B) ____________, or collect a (C)____________ from an inpatient who is not (D) ____________ an ID band.
2. *Never* collect a (A) ____________ without some way to positively (B) ____________ that specimen to the (C) ____________.
3. *Do not* use veins on the (A) ____________ of the wrist because (B) ____________ lie close to the (C) ____________ in this area and can be easily injured.
4. Remember, a patient has the (A) ____________ to (B) ____________ testing.
5. For safety reasons, *do not* use a two-(A)____________ technique (also called the (B)____________) hold in which the entry point of the vein is (C) ____________ by the (D) ____________ finger above and the (E) ____________ below.
6. If the (A) ____________ end of the tube fills first, blood in the tube is in contact with the (B) ____________ and (C) ____________ can occur if there is a change in (D) ____________ in the patient's vein.
7. Laboratory personnel will assume that blood in (A) ____________ is capillary blood. If (B) ____________ blood is placed in a (C) ____________, it is important to label the specimen as (D) ____________ blood because reference ranges for some tests differ depending on the (E) ____________ of the specimen.
8. When identifying a patient *never* say, for example, (A) "____________ ____________ Mrs. Smith?" A person who is very (B) ____________, hard of hearing, or (C) ____________ may (D) ____________ "____________" to anything.
9. A phlebotomist must be able to recognize a (A) ____________ to avoid damaging the area, as it is a (B) ____________ patient's (C) ____________.
10. *Never* attempt to collect a blood specimen from a (A) ____________ patient. Such an attempt may (B) ____________ the patient and cause (C) ____________ to the patient or the phlebotomist.
11. Never use force to (A) ____________ a patient's arm or open a (B) ____________, as it can cause pain and (C) ____________.
12. An (A) ____________ patient may be able to feel (B) ____________ and (C) ____________ when you (D) ____________ the needle.
13. A common (A) ____________ and one that is irritating to the (B) ____________ impaired is to (C) ____________ your voice when you are speaking to them.
14. (A) ____________ births present an increased risk of (B) ____________ error.
15. (A) ____________ a crying child as soon as possible, because the (B) ____________ of crying and struggling can (C) ____________ blood components and lead to (D) ____________ test results.

KNOWLEDGE DRILL 8-2: SCRAMBLED WORDS

Unscramble the following words using the hints given in parenthesis. Write the correct spelling of the scrambled word on the line next to it.

1. cnirtoccen CONCENTRIC (with a common center)
2. cutecite UTECTIC (easily melted)
3. cyanept PATENCY (required of a vein before a draw)
4. darictipe PEDIATRIC (pertaining to children)
5. gnistaf FASTING (testing requirement)
6. hipabo PHOBIA (intense fear)
7. leaptap PALPATE (a way to examine a vein)
8. narcho ANCHOR (firmly secure)
9. pheosic HOSPICE (terminal care)
10. scenicaso ACCESSION (record in order)
11. striniequio REQUISITION (required order)
12. triecagri GERIATRIC (aged)

KNOWLEDGE DRILL 8-3: COMMON TEST STATUS DESIGNATIONS (text Table 8-1)

Fill in the blanks with the missing information.

Status	Meaning	When Used	Collection Conditions	Test Examples	Priority
(1) ______	Immediately (from Latin *statim*)	Test results are urgently needed on critical patients.	Immediately collect, test, and report results. Alert lab staff when (2) ______. ER stats typically have priority over other stats	Glucose (3) ______ Electrolytes Cardiac enzymes	First
Med Emerg	Medical Emergency (replaces stat)	Same as stat	Same as stat	Same as stat	(4) ______
Timed	Collect at a specific time	Tests for which timing is critical for accurate (5) ______	Collect as close as possible to requested time. (6) ______ actual time collected	2-hour PP (7) ______ Cortisol Cardiac enzymes (8) ______ Blood cultures	Second

(9) ______	As soon as possible	Test results are needed soon to respond to a (10) ______ situation, but patient is not critical.	Follow hospital protocol for type of test	Electrolytes Glucose H&H	(11) ______ or third depending on test
Fasting	No (12) ______ or drink except water for 8–12 hours prior to specimen collection	To eliminate diet effects on test results.	Verify that patient has fasted. If patient has not fasted, check to see if specimen should still be collected.	(13) ______ Cholesterol Triglycerides	(14) ______
NPO	Nothing by (15) ______ (From Latin *nil per os*)	Prior to surgery or other anesthesia procedures.	Do not give patient food or (16) ______ Refer requests to physician or nurse.	N/A	N/A
(17) ______	Before an operation	To determine patient eligibility for (18) ______.	Collect before the patient goes to surgery.	CBC, PTT, Platelet function studies	Same as (19) ______
Postop	After an operation	To assess patient condition after surgery.	Collect when patient is out of surgery.	(20) ______	Same as (21) ______
(22) ______	Relating to established procedure	Used to establish a diagnosis or monitor a patient's progress.	Collect in a timely manner but no urgency involved. Typically collected on morning sweeps or the next scheduled sweep.	CBC (24) ______ ______	(23) ______

KNOWLEDGE DRILL 8-4: TOURNIQUET RATIONALE

Answer the following questions in the space provided.

1. What does a tourniquet do and why is it needed in venipuncture procedures?

   IT CUTS OFF FLOW TO MAKE THE VEINS VISIABLE

2. Why is a tourniquet placed 3 to 4 inches above the intended venipuncture site?

   IT WILL COLLAPSES THE VEIN, AND LOOSES PURPOSE

3. Where is the tourniquet placed in drawing blood from a hand vein?

   ABOVE THE WRIST BONES 3INCHES ABOVE

4. What happens if too much tension is applied in fastening a tourniquet?

   YOU CAN PHYSICALLY HURT THE PATIENT AND CAUSE BRUSING., VEIN WILL COLLAPSE

5. What is the purpose of the loop created during tourniquet application?

   TO HELP IT EASIER TO GET OFF, RELEASE THE TOURNAQUET ONE HANDED.

6. Why is it important to release the tourniquet within 1 minute of application?

   BRUISING., AVOID. CHANGES COMPOSITION OF BLOOD.

KNOWLEDGE DRILL 8-5: GERIATRIC CHALLENGES

The text lists five challenges associated with collecting specimens from geriatric patients. One is "Effects of disease." Identify the four other challenges, describe how each can affect the specimen collection process, and explain how you would handle each one.

1. Challenge: ______________________

   Effect: ______________________

   How to handle: ______________________

2. Challenge:

   Effect:

   How to handle:

3. Challenge:

   Effect:

   How to handle:

4. Challenge:

   Effect:

   How to handle:

Skills Drills

SKILLS DRILL 8-1: REQUISITION ACTIVITY (Text Fig. 8-2)

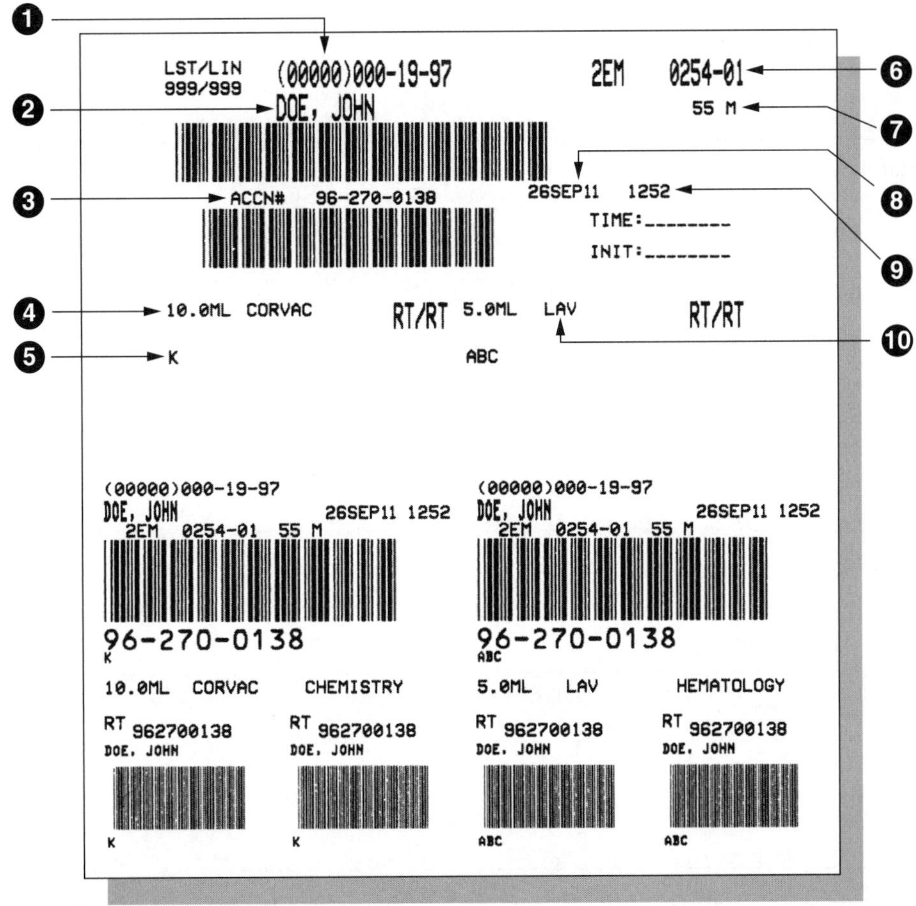
LST/LIN
999/999
(00000)000-19-97
2EM 0254-01
DOE, JOHN
55 M
ACCN# 96-270-0138
26SEP11 1252
TIME:________
INIT:________
10.0ML CORVAC
RT/RT
5.0ML LAV
RT/RT
K
ABC
(00000)000-19-97
DOE, JOHN
26SEP11 1252
2EM 0254-01 55 M
96-270-0138
K
(00000)000-19-97
DOE, JOHN
26SEP11 1252
2EM 0254-01 55 M
96-270-0138
ABC
10.0ML CORVAC
CHEMISTRY
5.0ML LAV
HEMATOLOGY
RT 962700138
DOE, JOHN
K
RT 962700138
DOE, JOHN
K
RT 962700138
DOE, JOHN
ABC
RT 962700138
DOE, JOHN
ABC

Identify each numbered item on the requisition and write the answer on the corresponding line below.

1. ______________________
2. ______________________
3. ______________________
4. ______________________
5. ______________________
6. ______________________
7. ______________________
8. ______________________
9. ______________________
10. ______________________

SKILLS DRILL 8-2: WORD BUILDING

Divide each word into all of its elements; preface (P), word root (WR), combining vowel (CV) and suffix (S). Write the word part, its definition, and the general meaning of the word on the corresponding lines. If the word does not have a particular word part, write NA (not applicable) in its place.

Example: geriatric

Elements ______*ger*______ / ______*iatr*______ / ___*ic*___
P WR S

Definitions ______*seniors*______ / ______*treatment*______ / ______ / ______*pertaining to*______

Meaning: pertaining to the treatment of the seniors

1. hemolysis

Elements ______________ / ______________ / ______ / ______________
P WR CV S

Definitions ______________ / ______________ / ______ / ______________

General Meaning:

2. antecubital

Elements ______________ / ______________ / ______ / ______________
P WR CV S

Definitions ______________ / ______________ / ______ / ______________

Meaning:

3. subcutaneous

Elements ______________ / ______________ / ______ / ______________
P WR CV S

Definitions ______________ / ______________ / ______ / ______________

Meaning:

4. hemodialysis

Elements ______________ / ______________ / ______ / ______________ / ______________
P WR CV WR S

Definitions ______________ / ______________ / ______ / ______________ / ______________

Meaning:

5. venous

Elements ______________ / ______________ / ______ / ______________
P WR CV S

Definitions ______________ / ______________ / ______ / ______________

Meaning:

6. pulmonary

Elements ______________ / ______________ / ______ / ______________
P WR CV S

Definitions ______________ / ______________ / ______ / ______________

General Meaning:

SKILLS DRILL 8-3: ROUTINE ETS VENIPUNCTURE (Text Procedure 8-2)

Fill in the blanks with the missing information.

Steps	Explanation/Rationale
1. Review and (1) ______________ the test request.	A test request is reviewed for completeness, date, and time of collection, status, and priority. The (2) ______________ process records the request and assigns it a (3) ______________ number used to (4) ______________ the specimen, related processes, and paperwork.
2. Approach, (5) ______________, and prepare patient.	The right approach for a successful patient encounter includes a professional bedside manner, being organized and efficient, and looking for signs that convey important inpatient information or infection-control precautions. Correct (6) ______________ is vital to patient safety and meaningful test results. Name, DOB and MR number must be verified and matched to the test order and inpatient's ID band. Preparing the patient by explaining procedures and addressing inquiries helps reduce patient anxiety.
3. Verify (7) ______________ restrictions and latex sensitivity.	Test results can be meaningless or (8) ______________ and patient care (9) ______________ if diet requirements have not been met. In such cases, consult the physician or nurse before proceeding. Exposure to latex can trigger a life-threatening reaction in those allergic to it, so it is vital that no latex items be used on a latex-sensitive patient or even brought into the room.
4. Sanitize (10) ______________.	Proper (11) ______________ ______________ plays a major role in infection control by protecting the phlebotomist, patient, and others from contamination. Gloves are sometimes put on at this point. Follow facility protocol.
5. Position patient, apply tourniquet, and ask patient to make a (12) ______________.	Proper positioning is important to patient comfort and venipuncture success. Place the patient's arm downward in a straight line from shoulder to wrist to aid in vein selection and avoid reflux as tubes are filled. A tourniquet placed 3–4 in. above the antecubital area enlarges veins and makes them easier to see, feel, and enter with a needle. A (13) ______________ fist makes the veins easier to see and feel and helps keep them from rolling.

6. Select vein, (14) ____________ ____________, ask patient to open fist.

Select a large, well-anchored vein. The median cubital should be the first choice, followed by the cephalic. The (15) ____________ should not be chosen unless no other vein is more prominent in either arm. Releasing the tourniquet and opening the fist helps prevent hemoconcentration.

7. Clean and (16) ____________ site.

Cleaning the site with an antiseptic such as 70% isopropyl alcohol helps avoid contaminating the specimen or patient with skin-surface bacteria picked up by the needle during venipuncture. Letting the site (17) ____________ naturally permits maximum antiseptic action, prevents contamination caused by wiping, and avoids stinging on needle entry and specimen hemolysis from residual alcohol.

8. Prepare equipment and put on (18) ____________.

Selecting appropriate equipment for the size, condition, and location of the vein is easier after vein selection. Preparing it while the site is drying saves time. Attach a needle to an ETS holder. Put the first tube in the holder now (see step 10) or wait until after needle entry. According to the OSHA BBP standard, (19) ____________ must be worn during phlebotomy procedures.

9. Reapply tourniquet, uncap and (20) ____________ needle.

The tourniquet aids needle entry. Pick up the tube holder with your dominant hand, placing your thumb on top near the needle end and fingers underneath. Uncap and (21) ____________ the needle for (22) ____________, and discard it if flawed.

10. Ask patient to remake a fist, (23) ____________ vein, and insert needle.

The fist aids needle entry. (24) ____________ stretches the skin, so the needle enters (25) ____________ and with less pain, and keeps the vein from rolling. Anchor by grasping the arm just below the elbow, supporting the back of it with your fingers. Place your thumb 1–2 in. below and slightly beside the vein and pull the skin toward the wrist.

Warn the patient. Line the needle up with the vein and insert it into the skin using a smooth forward motion. Stop when you feel a decrease in (26) ____________, often described as a "pop," and press your fingers into the arm to anchor the holder.

11. Establish blood flow, release (27) ____________, ask patient to open fist.	Blood will not flow until the needle pierces the tube stopper. Place a tube in the holder and push it partway onto the needle with a clockwise twist. Grasp the holder's flanges with your middle and index fingers, pulling back slightly to keep the holder from moving, and push the tube onto the needle with your thumb. Releasing the (28) ____________ and opening the fist allows blood flow to normalize (see step 6). According to CLSI standards, the tourniquet should be released as soon as possible after blood begins to flow and should not be left on longer than 1 minute.
12. Fill, remove, and (29) __________ __________ in order of draw.	Fill additive tubes until the vacuum is exhausted to ensure correct blood-to-additive ratio, and mix them (30) ____________ upon removal from the holder using 3 to 8 gentle inversions (depending on type and manufacturer) to prevent clot formation. Follow the CLSI order of draw to prevent additive carryover between tubes.
13. Place gauze, remove needle, activate (31) ____________ feature, and apply pressure.	A clean, folded gauze square is placed over the site so pressure can be applied immediately after needle removal. Remove the needle in one smooth motion without lifting up or pressing down on it. Immediately apply pressure to the site with your free hand while simultaneously activating the needle (32) ____________ with the other to prevent the chance of a needlestick.
14. Discard (33) ____________ ____________.	According to OSHA, the needle and the (34) ____________ ____________ must go into the sharps container as a unit because removing a needle from the holder exposes the user to sharps injury.
15. (35) ____________ ____________.	To avoid mislabeling errors, label tubes before leaving the (36) ____________ or dismissing the patient.
16. Observe special (37) ____________ instructions.	For accurate results, some specimens require special (38) ____________ such as cooling in crushed ice (e.g., ammonia), transportation at (39) ____________ temperature (e.g., cold agglutinin), or protection from (40) ____________ (e.g., bilirubin).

17. Check (41) ____________ ____________ and apply bandage

The patient's arm must be examined to verify that (42) ____________ has stopped. Just because bleeding has stopped on the skin surface does not mean that the site has stopped bleeding from the vein. The site must be checked for signs of bleeding beneath the skin. If bleeding persists beyond 5 minutes, notify the patient's nurse or physician. If bleeding has stopped, apply a bandage and advise the patient to keep it in place for at least 15 minutes.

18. Dispose of used and (43) ____________ ____________ materials.

Materials such as needle caps and wrappers are normally discarded in the regular trash. Some facilities require that contaminated items such as blood-soaked gauze be discarded in (44) ____________ containers.

19. Thank patient, remove gloves, and (45) ____________.

Thanking the patient is courteous and professional. Gloves must be removed in an aseptic manner and hands washed or (46) ____________ with hand sanitizer as an infection-control precaution.

20. (47) ____________ ____________.

Prompt delivery to the lab protects specimen (48) ____________ and is typically achieved by personal delivery, transportation via a pneumatic tube system, or by a courier service.

SKILLS DRILL 8-4: USING A SYRINGE TRANSFER DEVICE (Text Procedure 8-5)

Fill in the blanks with the missing information.

Steps	Explanation/Rationale
1. Remove the (1) ____________ from the syringe and discard it in a sharps container.	The (2) ____________ must be removed to attach the transfer device.
2. Attach the syringe (3) __________ to the transfer device hub, rotating it to ensure secure attachment.	Secure attachment is necessary to prevent (4) ________ ________ during transfer.
3. Hold the syringe (5) ____________ with the tip down and the transfer device at the bottom.	This ensures (6) ____________ placement of tubes to prevent (7) ____________ ____________.
4. Place an ETS tube in the barrel of the transfer device and push it all the way (8) __________.	The device has an internal (9) ____________ that will puncture the stopper and allow blood to flow into the tube.
5. Follow the (10) ________ ________ ________ if multiple tubes are to be filled.	The (11) ________ ________ ________ is designed to prevent (12) ________ ________ between tubes.
6. Keep the tubes and transfer device (13) ____________.	This ensures that tubes fill from bottom to (14) __________, preventing additive (15) ____________ with the needle and (16) ______________ of subsequent tubes.

7. Let tubes fill using the (17) ____________ draw of the tube. Do not push on the (18) ____________ ____________.	Forcing blood into a tube by pushing the (19) ____________ can (20) ____________ the specimen or cause the tube stopper to pop off, splashing tube contents.
8. If you must underfill a tube, (21) ____________ ____________ to stop blood flow before removing it.	Tubes quickly fill until the (22) ____________ is gone. (23) ____________ stops the tube from filling.
9. (24) ________ additive tubes as soon as they are removed.	(25) ____________ tubes must be mixed (26) ____________ for proper (27) ____________, including preventing (28) ____________ formation in anticoagulant tubes.
10. When finished, discard the syringe and transfer device (29) ____________ in a sharps container.	Removing the (30) ____________ from the syringe would expose the user to (31) ____________ in the hubs of both units. The transfer device must go into the sharps because of its internal (32) ____________.

SKILLS DRILL 8-5: HIGHLIGHTS OF HAND VENIPUNCTURE PROCEDURE (Text Procedure 8-3)

The following are highlights from the procedure for venipuncture of a hand vein using a butterfly and ETS holder. Fill in the blanks with the missing information.

1. Position Hand: Support the (A) ____________ on the (B) ____________ or armrest. Have the patient (C) ____________ the fingers slightly or make a fist.
2. Select Vein: Select a vein that has (A) ____________ or resilience and can be easily (B) ____________. Wiping the hand with (C) ____________ sometimes makes the veins more (D) ____________.
3. Prepare Equipment: Attach the butterfly to an (A) ____________. Grasp the (B) ____________ near the needle end and run your fingers down its length, (C) ____________ it slightly to help keep it from (D) ____________.
4. Uncap and Inspect Needle: Hold the (A) ____________ portion of the butterfly between your (B) ____________ and index finger or fold the wings upright and grasp them together. Cradle the tubing and holder in the (C) ____________ of your dominant hand or lay it next to the patient's hand. Uncap and inspect the needle for (D) ____________ and discard if flawed.
5. Anchor Vein: To anchor, use your (A) ____________ hand to hold the patient's hand just below the (B) ____________ and pull the skin taut over the (C) ____________ with your thumb while (D) ____________ the patient's fingers.
6. Insert the Needle: Insert the needle into the vein at a shallow angle between (A)____________ degrees. A (B) "____________" or small amount of (C) ____________ will appear in (D) ____________ when the needle is in the vein. "Seat" the needle by slightly threading it within the (E) ____________ of the vein to keep it from twisting back out of the vein if you let go of it.
7. Establish Blood Flow: The (A) ____________ of blood in the (B) ____________ indicates vein (C) ____________. Blood will not flow until the needle pierces the tube (D)____________. Place a tube in the holder and push it part way onto the needle with a clockwise twist. Grasp the holder (E) ____________ with your middle and index fingers, pulling back slightly to keep the (F) ____________ from moving, and push the tube onto the needle with your thumb.
8. Fill, Remove, and Mix Tubes: Maintain tubing and holder (A) ____________ the site, and positioned so that the tubes fill from the (B) ____________ ____________ to prevent (C) ____________.

SKILLS DRILL 8-6: HIGHLIGHTS OF NEEDLE-AND-SYRINGE VENIPUNCTURE PROCEDURE (Text Procedure 8-4)

The following are highlights from the needle-and-syringe venipuncture procedure. Fill in the blanks with the missing information.

1. Prepare Equipment: It is easier to select (A) ____________ equipment after the (B) ____________ has been chosen. Preparing it while the site is (C) ____________ saves time.
2. Uncap and Inspect Needle: Hold the syringe in your dominant hand as you would an (A) ____________. Place your (B) ____________ on top near the needle end and fingers underneath. Uncap and (C) ____________ the needle for defects and discard it if flawed.
3. Establish Blood Flow: Establishment of blood flow is normally indicated by (A) ____________ in the (B) ____________ of the syringe. In some cases blood will not flow until the syringe (C) ____________ is (D) ____________ ____________.
4. Fill Syringe: Venous blood will not automatically (A)____________ a syringe. It must be filled by slowly pulling back on the (B) ____________ with your free hand. Steady the syringe as you would an (C) ____________ during routine venipuncture.
5. Discard Needle: The needle must be removed and discarded in the sharps container so that a (A) ____________ ____________ for (B) ____________ the tubes can be (C) ____________ to the syringe. A (D) ____________ ____________ greatly reduces the chance of accidental (E) ____________ and confines any (F) ____________ or spraying that may be generated as the tube is removed.

Crossword

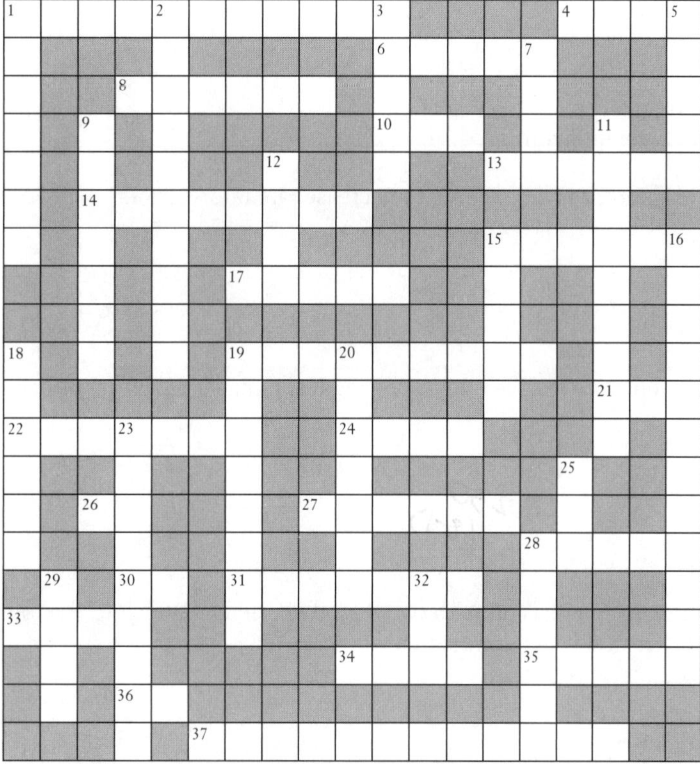

ACROSS

1. Meaning of AC
4. Order stating not to revive (plural)
6. Preferred is 30 degrees or less
8. To secure firmly by pulling the skin taut
10. Closed blood collection system (abbrev.)
13. Applied to sample tube after collection, never before (plural)
14. To use an alcohol-based cleansing solution
15. Pertaining to veins or blood passing through them
17. Median cutaneous ___________
19. Alcohol used in routine venipuncture
21. Intensive care unit (abbrev.)
22. Vein status that requires the use of small-gauge needle and syringe
24. Pulled tight
26. Assigned number to each patient (abbrev.)
27. Equipment checked for imperfections/burrs before puncturing
28. Used instead of cotton ball over the puncture hole
30. Location of preferred choice of veins for venipuncture (abbrev.)
31. State of not eating
33. Tight hand used to stabilize veins in the arm
34. To thread the needle within the lumen
35. Basilic and cephalic
36. Identification (abbrev.)
37. Type of dialysis

DOWN

1. Another name for ID bracelet
2. Proper way to swipe a swab to clean the site
3. Type of glove and tourniquet responsible for allergenic reactions
5. Used to relay patient status and usually posted on the door (plural)
7. Topical anesthetic applied to skin to ease puncture pain
9. Type of care for patients who are terminally ill
11. Pink- to red-colored plasma is due to ___________
12. Point at which the needle will enter the vein
15. Type of gloves used for venipuncture
16. Layer of connective and adipose tissue below the dermis
18. Backflow of blood from collection tube to patient's vein
19. The most important part of venipuncture procedure is to ___________ the patient
20. One who is receiving medical care
23. Pertaining to elderly patients
25. Test commonly ordered on geriatric patients if RA is suspected (abbrev.)
28. Nitrile or vinyl ___________
29. Prescribed course of eating and drinking
32. National Institute on Aging (abbrev.)

Chapter Review Questions

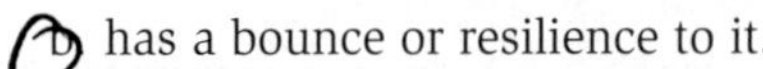

1. A vein that has patency:
   a. feels hard and cord-like.
   b. has a bounce or resilience to it.
   c. is fairly deep in the tissues.
   d. should not be used for venipuncture.

2. Which type of test requisition has been shown to decrease laboratory errors?
   a. Bar coded
   b. Computer
   c. Manual
   d. Verbal

3. The time is 0750 hours. You have received the following test requests on different patients. Which test specimen should you collect first?
   a. CBC ordered ASAP
   b. Cortisol ordered for 0800
   c. Fasting glucose
   d. Postop hemoglobin

4. A student asks the patient for permission to draw a blood specimen. Which of the following answers implies that the student does not really have permission?
   a. As long as you're good at it.
   b. Which arm do you want?
   c. Yes, but I would rather not.
   d. All of the above.

5. You have a request to collect a stat specimen. A doctor is with the patient when you arrive. What should you do?
   a. Call your supervisor and ask what you should do.
   b. Excuse yourself and politely ask the doctor for permission to do the draw.
   c. Leave the room and return when the doctor is gone.
   d. Stand there quietly until the doctor notices you and asks you what you want.

6. You are in the process of identifying an inpatient. The patient's verbal confirmation of name and date of birth matches the requisition, but the medical record number is different. What should you do?
   a. Change the requisition number to match the ID band and collect the specimen.
   b. Collect the specimen and inform the patient's nurse that the ID needs correcting.
   c. Do not collect the specimen until the problem has been addressed and resolved.
   d. Fill out an incident report and return to the lab without collecting the specimen.

7. You are a phlebotomy student on rotation at an outpatient site. A patient who seems extremely apprehensive about having her blood drawn tells you that she is afraid of needles. What should you do?
   a. Ask an experienced phlebotomist to perform the draw for you.
   b. Explain to her that you will use a small needle that barely hurts.
   c. Tell her that it is not a big deal and that she shouldn't be afraid.
   d. Use an ice pack to numb the site before drawing the specimen.

8. There are two patients in a room. One of them has a latex allergy. You have a request to collect a blood specimen on the other one. How should you proceed?
   a. Ask the allergic patient to wear a mask until you leave.
   b. Do not take anything that contains latex into the room.
   c. Pull the curtain between the beds and proceed normally.
   d. Your patient is not allergic to latex, so proceed as usual.

9. The best way to judge patency of a vein is to:
   a. feel it to determine the strength of the pulse.
   b. palpate above and below where you first feel it.
   c. press and release it several times to determine resilience.
   d. roll your finger from side to side while pressing against it.

10. Which of the following statements describes proper venipuncture technique?
   a. Clean the site quickly while the tourniquet is on.
   b. Fill additive tubes until the vacuum is exhausted.
   c. Keep the tourniquet on until the last tube is full.
   d. Wipe the alcohol dry to prevent it from stinging.

11. What is the most critical error a phlebotomist can make?
   a. Collecting a timed specimen late
   b. Failing to collect a specimen
   c. Giving a patient a hematoma
   d. Misidentifying a patient specimen

12. Which needle can be removed from the blood collection unit before disposal?
   a. Butterfly needle
   b. ETS needle
   c. Syringe needle
   d. None of the above

13. When should additive tubes be mixed?
   a. After all the other tubes have been collected.
   b. As soon as they are removed from the holder.
   c. Never. Additive tubes do not require mixing.
   d. While you are filling any of the other tubes.

14. You have made two unsuccessful attempts while trying to collect an ASAP specimen on an inpatient. The specimen cannot be collected by skin puncture. What should you do next?
   a. Ask another phlebotomist to collect it.
   b. Ask the patient's nurse to do the draw.
   c. Collect it by arterial puncture.
   d. Try to draw it one more time.

15. The proper way to transfer blood from a syringe into an ETS tube is to:
   a. discard the needle, open the tube, and slowly eject the blood into it.
   b. hold the tube carefully and insert the needle through the tube stopper.
   c. place the tube in a rack and insert the needle through the tube stopper.
   d. safely remove the needle and attach a transfer device to fill the tube.

16. How can you tell that you are in a vein when drawing blood with a butterfly?
   a. Engage the tube to see if it will fill.
   b. Blood usually appears in the tubing.
   c. You can hear a soft popping sound.
   d. There is no easy way you can tell.

17. You are performing a venipuncture on a difficult vein using a butterfly. You have an SST and a light blue–topped tube to collect. How do you proceed?
   a. Collect and mix the SST before filling and mixing the light-blue top.
   b. Collect and mix the light-blue top before filling and mixing the SST.
   c. Draw a clear tube, fill and mix the light-blue top, then fill and mix the SST.
   d. Draw half the SST, then fill and mix the light-blue top, then finish the SST.

18. Interventions to ease pain in collecting blood specimens from infants include:
    a. EMLA.
    b. oral sucrose.
    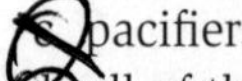
    c. pacifiers.
    d. all of the above.

19. Skin changes in elderly patients can make it harder to:
    a. anchor veins.
    b. injure veins.
    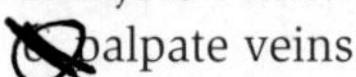
    c. palpate veins.
    d. see the veins.

20. Which type of disease is most likely to cause tremors?
    a. Alzheimer's
    b. Arthritis
    c. Diabetes
    d. Parkinson's

CASE STUDIES

Case Study 8-1 Patient ID and Specimen Labeling

A phlebotomist received a verbal request for a stat blood draw in the ER. When he arrived the nurse told him that the patient (Mr. Johnson) was in bed 1 and needed electrolytes and an H&H drawn. The patient had no ID band. The nurse assured the phlebotomist that it was the correct patient and that she would prepare the requisition and labels while he drew the specimens. The patient was able to verbally confirm name and date of birth, so the phlebotomist proceeded to collect the specimens, a green top and a lavender top. Just as he was finishing up, the nurse told the phlebotomist that they had another stat draw in bed 3. This patient needed electrolytes and glucose specimens drawn. The nurse said that she hadn't had time to prepare the requisition or labels for either patient, but she would do so now. The phlebotomist put the first two specimens in his phlebotomy tray and headed for bed 3. This patient was unconscious, and no one else was there to confirm his identity. The nurse said she didn't know his name either, as he had no identification with him when he was found. The phlebotomist proceeded to collect the specimens, a green top and lavender top, as with the first patient. He put the specimens in the tray when he was finished and went to the nurses' station for the requisitions and labels, which the nurse did have ready for him. When he went to label the specimens he had to stop and think about which specimens were the correct ones for each patient, since they were the same type of tubes. He was pretty sure he had put each patient's specimens at opposite ends of the tray, but had he turned the tray around since then? He decided that the ones that felt warmest were the last ones drawn, placed the labels on the tubes, and delivered them to the lab.

QUESTIONS

1. The phlebotomist made several errors. What were they?
2. What should the phlebotomist have done differently to prevent each error?
3. How might the actions of the phlebotomist affect treatment of the patients?

Case Study 8-2 Blood Volume, Equipment Selection, and Syringe Transfer Technique

A phlebotomist must collect specimens for a PTT and a CBC on an infant. The infant is several months old but was born prematurely and weighs only 5 pounds. The phlebotomist is surprised to see that the infant has a prominent median cubital vein. He uses a 10-mL syringe and a 23-gauge butterfly needle and is able to collect about 5 mL of blood before the tiny vein blows and a hematoma starts to form. He withdraws the needle and quickly bandages the site. He uses a transfer device to deliver the required 4.5 mL into a light blue–top tube for the PTT. He then uses a 5-mL syringe to draw another 5-mL of blood from a vein in the infant's other arm. He then discovers that he does not have another transfer device, so he grabs the lavender top and attempts to insert the needle through the tube stopper. The needle slips and jabs his hand. He is bleeding badly, so he drops the tube and syringe into his phlebotomy tray and runs to the sink to wash the wound. He then wraps a paper towel around his hand and returns to fill the lavender-top tube. This time he removes the needle from the syringe and the stopper from the tube. He injects the blood into the tube and replaces the stopper. He labels both tubes and returns to the lab. Specimen processing ultimately rejects both specimens, the PTT because of hemolysis and the CBC because of clotting.

QUESTIONS

1. What is the infant's estimated blood volume and calculated blood volume? How many milliliters of blood would be 10% of each of these numbers?
2. Was it appropriate to collect 10 mL of blood from the infant for the two tests? Why or why not?
3. How could the phlebotomist have collected less blood for the required tests?
4. How could the phlebotomist have avoided injury?
5. What could have caused the hemolysis of the PTT and the clotting of the CBC?

(1) IT SHOULD BE 115 mL/kg

(2) NO, THE BABY ONLY WEIGHED 5lbs AND HE WAS ONLY SUPPOSE TO DRAW .23L

(3) BY CALCULATING THE AMOUNT SUPPOSE TO FIRST.

(4) BY BEING CAREFUL

(5)

CHAPTER 9

Preanalytical Considerations

OBJECTIVES

Study the information in your textbook that corresponds to each objective to prepare yourself for the activities in this chapter.

1. Define the key terms and abbreviations listed at the beginning of this chapter.
2. List and describe the physiological variables that influence laboratory test results and identify the tests most affected by each one.
3. List problem areas to avoid in site selection, identify causes for concern, and describe procedures to follow when encountering each.
4. Identify and describe various vascular access sites and devices and explain what to do when they are encountered.
5. Identify, describe, and explain how to handle patient complications associated with blood collection.
6. Identify, describe, and explain how to avoid or handle procedural errors, specimen quality concerns, and reasons for failure to draw blood.

Matching

Use choices only once unless otherwise indicated.

MATCHING 9-1: KEY TERMS AND DESCRIPTIONS

Match each key term with the *best* description.

Key Terms (1–17)

1. ______ A-line
2. ______ AV shunt/fistula/graft
3. ______ Basal state
4. ______ Bilirubin
5. ______ CVAD
6. ______ CVC
7. ______ Diurnal/circadian
8. ______ Edema
9. ______ Exsanguination
10. ______ Hematoma
11. ______ Hemoconcentration
12. ______ Hemolysis
13. ______ Hemolyzed
14. ______ Heparin/saline lock
15. ______ Iatrogenic
16. ______ Icteric
17. ______ IV

Descriptions (1–17)

A. Abnormal accumulation of fluid in the tissues
B. Blood loss to the point where life cannot be sustained
C. Catheter placed in an artery, most commonly the radial
D. Catheter with a stopcock or cap for delivering medication or drawing blood
E. Central vascular access device or indwelling line
F. Central venous catheter or central venous line
G. Decrease in blood fluid with an increase in nonfilterable components
H. Destruction of RBCs and release of hemoglobin into the serum or plasma
I. Happening daily, or having a 24-hour cycle
J. Product of the breakdown of RBCs
K. Resting metabolic state of the body early in the morning after a 12-hour fast
L. Surgical joining of an artery and vein
M. Swelling or mass of blood caused by blood leaking from a blood vessel
N. Term used to describe a specimen affected by hemolysis
O. Term used to describe a specimen marked by jaundice
P. Term used to describe an adverse condition due to the effects of treatment
Q. Within, or pertaining to the inside of a vein

Key Terms (18–33)

18. ______ Jaundice
19. ______ Lipemia
20. ______ Lipemic
21. ______ Lymphostasis
22. ______ Mastectomy
23. ______ Petechiae
24. ______ PICC
25. ______ Preanalytical
26. ______ Pre-examination
27. ______ Reference ranges
28. ______ Reflux

Descriptions (18–33)

A. Backflow of blood into the vein during venipuncture
B. Breast removal
C. Clotted, or denoting a vessel containing a clot
D. Condition of increased lipid content in the blood
E. Fainting
F. Hard, cord-like, and lacking resilience
G. Icterus, a condition characterized by increased bilirubin
H. Normal lab test values for healthy individuals
I. Peripherally inserted central catheter
J. Prior to analysis
K. Relating to the action of a particular nerve on blood vessels
L. Stagnation or stoppage of the normal blood flow
M. Stoppage or obstruction of normal lymph flow
N. Term used to describe serum or plasma that has a milky look
O. Tiny, nonraised red spots appearing on patient's skin
P. Word that means the same as preanalytical

29. ______ Sclerosed
30. ______ Syncope
31. ______ Thrombosed
32. ______ Vasovagal
33. ______ Venous stasis

MATCHING 9-2: PHYSIOLOGICAL EFFECT AND TEST

Match the physiological effect to the associated test.

Physiological Effect

1. ______ Crying can increase levels
2. ______ Decreases with age
3. ______ Dehydration increases levels
4. ______ Elevated levels are related to jaundice
5. ______ Fatty foods increase levels
6. ______ Fever causes levels to increase
7. ______ Increases with altitude
8. ______ Levels normally peak around 0800 hours
9. ______ Pancreatitis from steroid use increases levels
10. ______ Requires documentation of patient's position during collection
11. ______ Smoking decreases levels
12. ______ Stays elevated for 24 hours or more after exercise

Test

A. Amylase
B. Bilirubin
C. CK
D. Coagulation factors
E. Cortisol
F. Creatinine clearance
G. IGA
H. Insulin
I. Lipids
J. Plasma renin
K. RBC count
L. WBC count

MATCHING 9-3: PROBLEM SITE AND DRAWBACK

Match the problem venipuncture site to the possible drawback if a blood specimen is collected from it.

Problem Site

1. ______ Antecubital area with a large hematoma
2. ______ Edematous arm
3. ______ Mastectomy on that side of the body
4. ______ Obese arm
5. ______ Recently burned antecubital area
6. ______ Tattoo-covered arm
7. ______ Vein that feels sclerosed

Drawback

A. Could mean veins are deeper than normal.
B. Dyes might interfere with testing.
C. Impaired circulation could affect test results.
D. Results could be erroneous due to lymphostasis.
E. Site may be painful and susceptible to infection.
F. Skin could be injured by tourniquet application.
G. Specimen could be contaminated by hemolyzed blood.

MATCHING 9-4: SCENARIOS AND VASCULAR ACCESS DEVICES

Match the type of equipment described in the following scenarios with the list of vascular access devices.

Scenarios

1. ______ A nurse is collecting a blood gas specimen from tubing inserted in the underside of a patient's left wrist on the thumb side.
2. ______ A nurse is palpating an area in the patient's upper chest. She tells the patient that she is looking for the "chamber."
3. ______ A patient in the dialysis unit has what appears to be a loop under the skin on the inside of his forearm in which the large needles connected to the dialysis tubing have been inserted.
4. ______ There are several short lengths of capped tubing protruding from a patient's left arm, just above the antecubital area.
5. ______ There is a device inserted on the back of a patient's arm just above the wrist. The device has a thin, rubber-like cover through which a nurse is administering fluid from a syringe.
6. ______ The patient is a line draw. He has three short lengths of capped tubing protruding from his chest. The nurse draws the specimen for you from one of the lengths of tubing.

Vascular Access Devices

A. Arterial line (A-line)
B. Arteriovenous (AV) shunt
C. Central venous catheter (CVC)
D. Heparin lock
E. Implanted port
F. Peripherally inserted central catheter (PICC)

MATCHING 9-5: RISK AND PROCEDURAL ERROR

Match the risk to the procedural error involved.

Risk

1. ____ Hematoma formation
2. ____ Iatrogenic anemia
3. ____ Inadvertent arterial puncture
4. ____ Infection
5. ____ Nerve damage
6. ____ Reflux
7. ____ Vein damage

Procedural Error

A. A patient is a difficult draw so the phlebotomist draws from the exact same site each time.
B. Blood fills the stopper end of the tube first.
C. Blood spurts into the tube after the needle is redirected multiple times.
D. The needle goes through the vein.
E. The patient complains of great pain during a missed attempt to draw from the basilic vein.
F. The phlebotomist always wipes the alcohol dry before performing a venipuncture.
G. Three 5-mL tubes of blood are drawn from an infant at one time.

MATCHING 9-6: SENTENCE BEGINNING AND ENDING

Match the beginning of the sentence concerning causes of hemolysis with the letter of the correct sentence ending.

Sentence Beginning

1. Drawing blood through a ____
2. Failure to wipe away the first drop of ____
3. Forceful aspiration of ____
4. Forcing the blood ____
5. Frothing of blood ____
6. Horizontal transport of ____
7. Mixing additive tubes ____
8. Partially filling a ____
9. Pulling back the ____
10. Rough handling ____
11. Squeezing the site ____
12. Syringe transfer ____
13. Using a large volume ____
14. Using a needle with a ____

Sentence Ending

A. blood during a syringe draw
B. capillary blood, which can contain alcohol residue
C. caused by improper fit of the needle on a syringe
D. delay in which partially clotted blood is forced into a tube
E. during capillary specimen collection
F. during transport
G. from a syringe into an evacuated tube
H. hematoma or from a vein with a hematoma
I. normal draw sodium fluoride tube
J. plunger too quickly during a syringe draw
K. too-small diameter for venipuncture
L. tube with a small-diameter butterfly needle
M. tubes, which lets the blood slosh back and forth
N. vigorously, shaking them, or inverting them too quickly or forcefully

Labeling Exercises

LABELING EXERCISE 9-1: IDENTIFYING VENIPUNCTURE PROBLEMS

One of the following illustrations shows correct needle position. The other illustrations depict venipuncture problems. Select the corrective action required for each illustration from the list below and write the letter of the corrective action on the corresponding line. Choices may be used more than once.

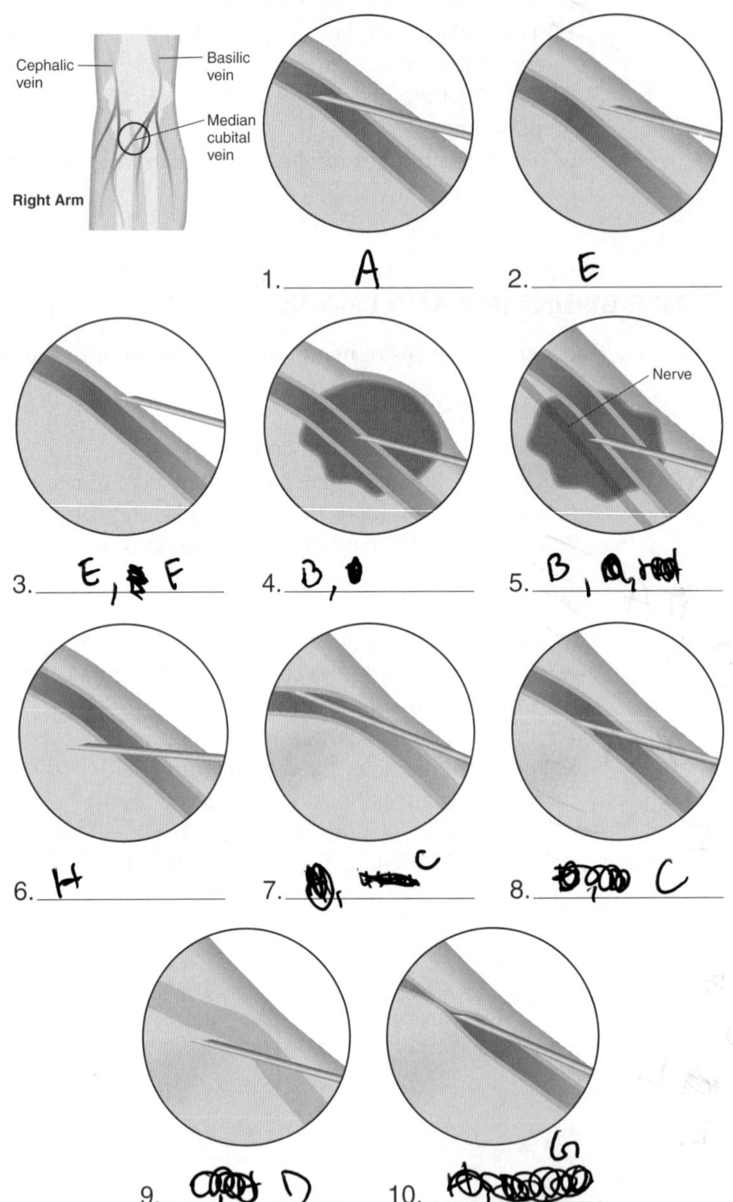

Corrective Action

A. Correct needle position; blood can flow freely—no action required.
B. Discontinue the draw.
C. Disengage the tube, pull the needle back slightly, and re-engage the tube.
D. Disengage the tube, pull the needle back until only the bevel is under the skin, anchor the vein, redirect the needle, and re-engage the tube.
E. Gently push the needle forward.
F. Put on a new tube.
G. Try using a smaller-volume tube.
H. Withdraw the needle slowly until blood flow is obtained.

LABELING EXERCISE 9-2: VAD IDENTIFICATION

The following are examples of VAD placement in patients. Identify and label each one by writing the type of VAD on the line beneath it. Use the VAD full name and initials if applicable.

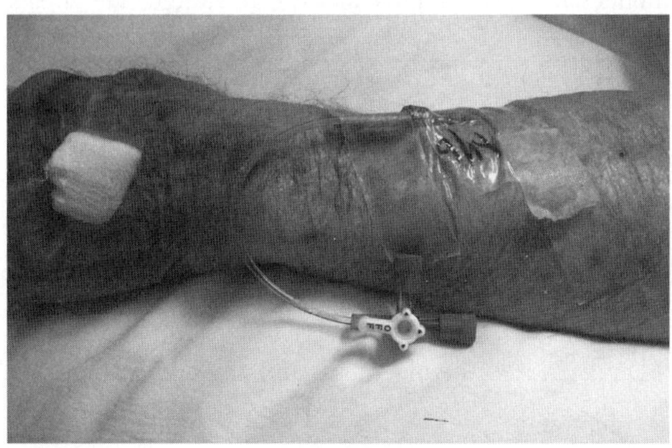

1. ______________________________

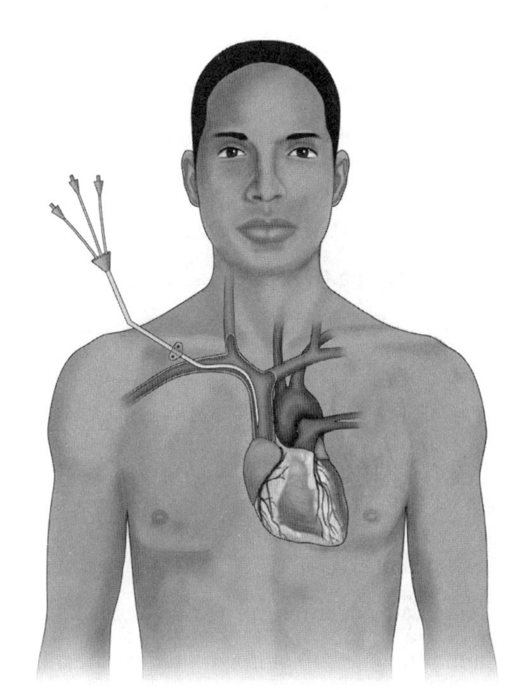

2. ______________________________

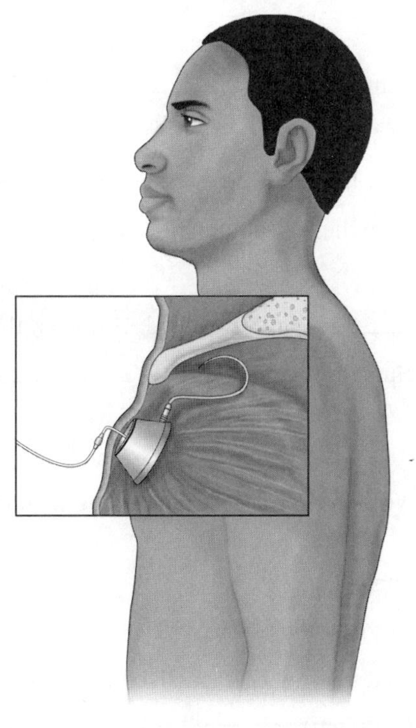

3. ______________________________

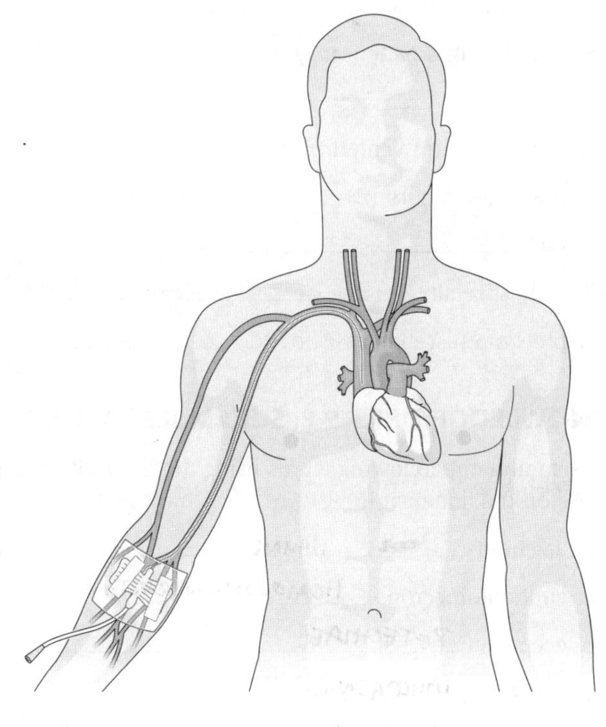

4. ______________________________

Knowledge Drills

KNOWLEDGE DRILL 9-1: CAUTION AND KEY POINT RECOGNITION

The following sentences are from caution and key point statements found throughout Chapter 9 of the textbook. Using the TEXTBOOK, fill in the blanks with the missing information.

1. The National Cholesterol Education Program recommends that (A) ____________ profiles be collected in a consistent manner after the patient has been either (B) ____________ ____________ or ____________ quietly for a minimum of (C) ____________.
2. Never apply a (A) ____________ ____________ ____________ or (B) ____________, or perform venipuncture, on an arm with a (C) ____________.
3. The use of (A) ____________ ____________ to revive patients who have fainted can have unwanted side effects such as (B) ____________________ distress in (C) ____________________ individuals and is not recommended.
4. If marked or (A) ____________ ____________ occurs, or the patient asks you to remove the (B) ____________ for any reason, the venipuncture should be (C) ____________________ immediately, even if there are no other signs of (D) ____________ ____________.
5. Extreme pain, a burning or (A) ____________-____________ sensation, (B) ____________ of the arm, and pain that radiates up or down the arm are all signs of (C) ____________ involvement, and any one of them requires immediate (D) ____________________ of the venipuncture.
6. Hand or fist (A) ____________________ can (B) ____________________ blood (C) ____________________ levels up to 20%.
7. (A) ____________________ is painful to the patient and can damage (B) ____________ or lead to inadvertent puncture of an (C) ____________.
8. Jaundice in a patient may indicate (A) ____________ inflammation caused by (B) ____________ B or C (C) ____________.
9. Never perform venipuncture through a (A) ____________________. If there is no alternative site, perform the venipuncture (B) ____________ to the (C) ____________ to ensure the collection of (D) ____________-____________ blood.
10. Only specially (A) ____________ personnel should access (B) ____________ to draw blood. However, the phlebotomist may assist by (C) ____________________ the specimen to the appropriate (D) ____________.

KNOWLEDGE DRILL 9-2: SCRAMBLED WORDS

Unscramble the following words using the hints given in parentheses. Write the correct spelling of the scrambled word on the line next to it.

1. ajecudin JAUNDICE (could indicate hepatitis)
2. cimhootninecronat HEMOCONCENTRATION (an indirect result of venous stasis)
3. ecepahiet PETECHIAE (a sign that the site may bleed excessively)
4. oratiecing IATROGENIC (as a result of treatment)
5. polsecdal COLLAPSED (describes a vein that has shut down)

6. psoynec SYNCOPE (patient reaction to fear of venipuncture)
7. rudalin DIAURNAL (happening daily)
8. sblaa BASAL (type of metabolic state)
9. smettmycoa MASECTOMY (issues with this side for a blood draw)
10. soyiteb OBESITY (could lead to difficult arm draws)
11. thrandeoyid DEHYDRATION (decrease in total body fluid)
12. xuferl REFLUX (arm position helps avoid this)

KNOWLEDGE DRILL 9-3: HEMATOMA FORMATION

The following are six situations that can trigger hematoma formation. Fill in the blanks with the missing information.

1. The vein is FRAGILE OR TOO SMALL for the needle size.
2. The needle penetrates ALL THE WAY THROUGH THE VEIN.
3. The needle is ONLY PARTLY INSERTED into the vein.
4. Excessive or BLIND PROBING is used to locate the vein.
5. The needle is removed while the WHILE THE TOURNAQUET IS STILL ON.
6. PRESSURE is not adequately applied following venipuncture.

KNOWLEDGE DRILL 9-4: IATROGENIC BLOOD LOSS

List four ways to minimize iatrogenic blood loss.

1. COORDINATE WITH PHYSICIANS TO MINIMIZE DRAWS OF PAITENT.
2. FOLLOW QUALITY ASSURANCE PROCEDURES TO MINIMIZE RE-DRAWS
3. COLLECT MINIMUM REQUIRED SPECIUM VOLUMES ESPECIALLY ON INFANTS
4. KEEP A LOG OF DRAWS

KNOWLEDGE DRILL 9-5: HEMOCONCENTRATION

Place a "C" in front of each sentence that describes an action that causes hemoconcentration. Place a "P" in front of each sentence that describes an action that prevents hemoconcentration.

1. C Allowing the patient to pump the fist
2. P Asking the patient to release the fist upon blood flow
3. P Choosing an appropriate patent vein
4. C Excessively massaging the area when locating a vein
5. C Redirecting the needle multiple times in search of a vein
6. P Releasing the tourniquet within 1 minute

KNOWLEDGE DRILL 9-6: SERUM APPEARANCE

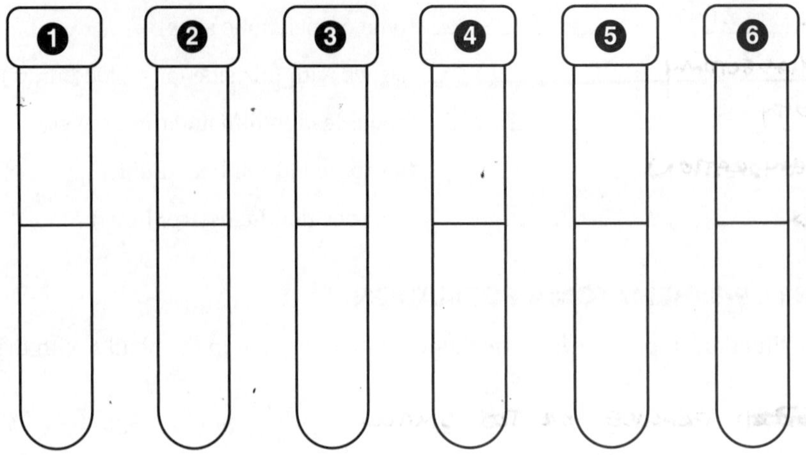

Color the serum in the numbered aliquot tubes according to the appearance listed by tube number below.

Serum Appearance

1. Icteric
2. Lipemic
3. Mild hemolysis
4. Moderate hemolysis
5. Gross hemolysis
6. Normal

Skills Drills

SKILLS DRILL 9-1: REQUISITION ACTIVITY

Instructions: Answer the following questions concerning the test requisition shown below.

1. Identify two physiological variables that affect Hgb levels. ______________________
2. If this patient's bilirubin level is high, how might it affect the patient's appearance? ______________________
3. How will the phlebotomist obtain this specimen? ______________________
4. Identify the tube required for each test. ______________________

Any Hospital USA
1123 West Physician Drive
Any Town USA

Laboratory Test Requisition

PATIENT INFORMATION:

Name: Smith (last) Jane (first) R (MI)

Identification Number: 09365784 Birth Date: 06/21/63

Referring Physician: Coleman

Date to be Collected: 03/11/2011 Time to be Collected: 0600

Special Instructions: Line draw only

TEST(S) REQUIRED:

____ NH4 – Ammonia	____ Gluc – glucose
X Bili – Bilirubin, total & direct	X Hgb – hemoglobin
____ BMP – basic metabolic panel	____ Lact – lactic acid/lactate
____ BUN - Blood urea nitrogen	____ Plt. Ct. – platelet count
____ Lytes – electrolytes	____ PT – prothrombin time
____ CBC – complete blood count	____ PTT – partial thromboplastin time
____ Chol – cholesterol	____ RPR – rapid plasma reagin
____ ESR – erythrocyte sed rate	____ T&S – type and screen
____ EtOH - alcohol	____ PSA – prostate specific antigen
____ D-dimer	Other ____________

SKILLS DRILL 9-2: WORD BUILDING

Divide each of the words below into all of its elements (parts); prefix (P), word root (WR), combining vowel (CV), and suffix (S). Write the word part, its definition, and the meaning of the word on the corresponding lines. If the word does not have a particular element, write NA (not applicable) in its place.

Example: Lymphostasis

	P	WR	CV	S
Elements		*lymph*	*o*	*stasis*
Definitions		*lymph*		*stopping*

Meaning: stopping lymph flow

1. Arteriovenous

	WR	CV	WR	S
Elements	ARTERI	O	VEN	OUS
Definitions	ARTERY		VEIN	PERTAINING TO

Meaning:

2. Hemolysis

	P	WR	CV	S
Elements		HEM	O	LYSIS
Definitions		BLOOD		BREAKDOWN

Meaning:

3. Intravenous

	P	WR	CV	S
Elements	INTRA	VEN		OUS
Definitions	WITHIN	VEIN		PERTAINING TOO

Meaning:

4. Lipemia

	P	WR	CV	S
Elements		LIP		EMIA
Definitions		FAT		BLOOD CONDITION

Meaning:

5. Sclerosis

	P	WR	CV	S
Elements		SCLER	[illegible]	OSIS
Definitions		HARD		CONDITION

Meaning:

6. Venostasis

	P	WR	CV	S
Elements		VEN	O	STASIS
Definitions		VEIN		STOPPING, CONTROLLING.

Meaning:

SKILLS DRILL 9-3: VENIPUNCTURE BELOW AN IV (text Procedure 9-1)

Fill in the blanks with the missing information.

Steps	Explanation/Rationale
1. Ask the patient's nurse to turn off the IV for at least (A) ______ prior to collection.	A phlebotomist is not qualified to (B) ______ IV ______. Turning off the IV for (C) ______ allows IV fluids to dissipate from the area.
2. Apply the tourniquet (D) ______ to the IV.	Avoids (E) ______ the IV.
3. Select a venipuncture site (F) ______ to the IV.	Venous blood flows (G) ______ ______. Drawing (H) ______ an IV affords the best chance of obtaining blood that is free of (I) ______.
4. Perform the venipuncture in a different (J) ______ if possible.	IV fluids can be present (K) ______ because of (L) ______ and may still be present after the IV is shut off because of poor venous circulation.
5. Ask the nurse to (M) ______ after the specimen has been collected.	IV flow rates must be (N) ______ and starting or adjusting them is not part of a phlebotomist's (O) ______.
6. Document that the specimen was collected (P) ______ an IV, indicate the (Q) ______ in the IV, and identify which (R) ______.	This aids (S) ______ and the patient's physician in the event that test (T) ______.

SKILLS DRILL 9-4: FAINTING PROCEDURE (text Procedure 9-2)

Fill in the blanks with the missing information.

Steps	Explanation/Rationale
1. Release the (A) ______________ and remove and discard the needle as quickly as possible.	Discontinuing the draw and discarding the needle protects the (B) ______________ from (C) __________ should the patient faint.
2. Apply pressure to the site while having the patient lower the (D) __________ and breathe deeply.	Pressure must be applied to prevent bleeding or bruising. Lowering the (E) __________ and breathing deeply helps get oxygenated blood to the (F) __________.
3. (G) __________ to the patient.	Diverts patient's attention, helps keep the patient (H) __________, and aids in assessing the patient's (I) ______________________.
4. Physically (J) __________ the patient.	Prevents (K) __________ in case of (L) __________.
5. Ask (M) ______________ and explain what you are doing if it is necessary to loosen a tight collar or tie.	Avoids (N) ______________ of actions that are (O) __________ __________ to hasten recovery.
6. Apply a (P) __________ compress or wet washcloth to the (Q) ______________ and ______________.	Part of the (R) __________ of __________.
7. Have someone stay with the patient until (S) __________ is complete.	Prevents patient from (T) __________ too soon and possibly causing (U) __________-__________.
8. Call (V) __________ personnel if the patient does not respond.	Emergency medicine is not in the phlebotomist's (W) __________ of __________.
9. (X) __________ the incident according to facility protocol.	(Y) __________ issues could arise and further (Z) ______________ is essential at that time.

Crossword

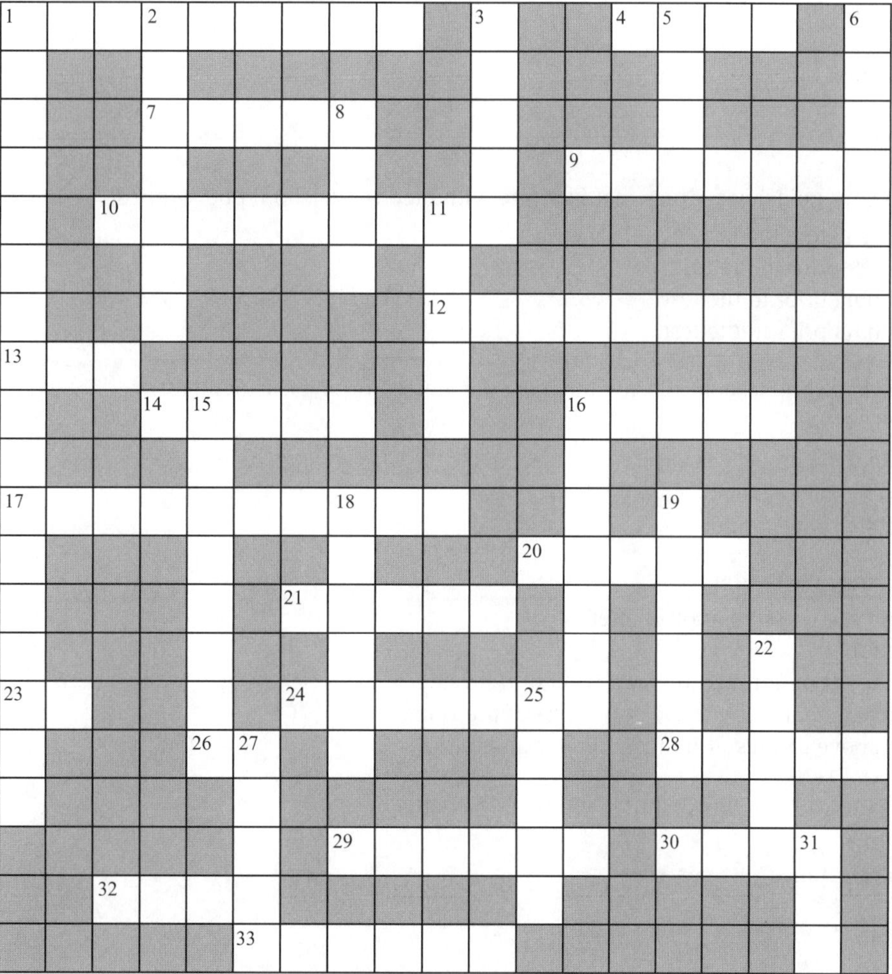

ACROSS

1. Result of damaged RBCs
4. Another name for indwelling line (abbrev.)
7. Possible result of mastectomy
9. Medical term for fainting
10. Having a 24-hour cycle
12. Describes blood loss due to testing
13. Broviac or Hickman (abbrev.)
14. Surgical connection of an artery and a vein
16. Excess tissue fluid
17. Describes a clotted vein
20. Increased temperature
21. Resting metabolic state
23. Intravenous line (abbrev.)
24. Fusion of an artery and a vein
26. Arteriovenous (abbrev.)
28. Trauma-related complication
29. Usually precedes vomiting
30. Preferred ______ is "fasting"
32. Phlebotomy national standards
33. Distinct buzzing VAD sensation

DOWN

1. Result of decreased plasma volume
2. Extreme chubbiness
3. Brand of elastic pressure wrap
5. Cephalic or basilic
6. Pertaining to increased bilirubin
8. Disease caused by HIV
11. Arterial line (abbrev.)
15. Most common phlebotomy complication
16. Causes turbid serum
18. Stagnation of fluid
19. Relating to a vein
22. To search for a vein
25. Can cause an allergic reaction
27. Can be the result of nausea
31. Value can change 50% from A.M. to P.M.

Chapter Review Questions

1. The medical term for fainting is:
   a. edematous.
   b. exsanguination.
   c. reflux.
   d. syncope.

2. According to CAP guidelines, drugs that interfere with blood tests should be stopped:
   a. 1 to 4 hours before the test.
   b. 4 to 24 hours prior to the test.
   c. 24 to 48 hours prior to the test.
   d. 48 to 72 hours prior to the test.

3. Which of the following tests is affected the most if collected from a crying infant?
   a. Bilirubin
   b. Cholesterol
   c. Lead level
   d. WBC count

4. A hematoma may result from:
   a. inadequate site pressure applied after a venipuncture.
   b. needle penetration through the back wall of the vein.
   c. using a needle that is too large for the size of the vein.
   d. All of the above can result in hematoma formation.

5. Results of this test have a direct correlation with the patient's age.
   a. Blood culture
   b. Creatinine clearance
   c. Glucose
   d. Hemoglobin

6. Which of the following specimen conditions would lead you to suspect that the patient was not fasting when it was collected?
   a. Cloudy white serum
   b. Pale-yellow plasma
   c. Pink to reddish plasma
   d. Yellowish brown serum

7. A phlebotomist needs to collect a plasma specimen for a coagulation test. The patient has an IV in the left arm near the wrist and a hematoma in the antecubital area of the right arm. Which of the following is the best place to collect the specimen?
   a. Above the IV
   b. From the IV after shutting it off for 2 minutes
   c. Distal to the hematoma
   d. All of the above are acceptable collection sites

8. A patient's arm is in anatomical position. There appears to be a loop under the skin between the wrist and the elbow. You feel a buzzing sensation when you touch it. What you are most likely feeling is a:
   a. AV graft.
   b. implanted port.
   c. PICC.
   d. sclerosed vein.

9. While you are in the middle of drawing a blood specimen, your patient starts to faint. The first thing you should do is:
   a. apply a cold compress directly to the patient's forehead.
   b. grab ammonia inhalant and wave it near the patient's nose.
   c. quickly release the tourniquet and remove the needle.
   d. tell the patient to lower the head and breathe deeply.

10. A patient has had a mastectomy on the left side and has an IV midway down the right arm. Where is the best place to perform a venipuncture?
   a. Above the IV on the right arm
   b. Below the IV on the right arm
   c. In the left antecubital area
   d. In the left hand or wrist

11. Blood loss to a point where life cannot be sustained is called:
   a. diurnal variation.
   b. exsanguination.
   c. iatrogenic anemia.
   d. vasovagal syncope.

12. Which of the following specimens would most likely be rejected for testing?
   a. A hemolyzed potassium specimen
   b. An icteric bilirubin specimen
   c. A nonfasting glucose specimen
   d. An underfilled serum tube

13. Which of the following is a clue that you have accidentally punctured an artery instead of a vein?
   a. The blood is dark bluish red.
   b. The blood spurts into the tube.
   c. The patient feels great pain.
   d. All of the above are clues.

14. The serum or plasma of a hemolyzed specimen would most likely look:
   a. cloudy or turbid.
   b. pale yellow.
   c. pinkish to red.
   d. yellowish brown.

15. Underfilling this tube will most likely result in a hemolyzed specimen.
   a. EDTA tube
   b. Light-blue top
   c. Gray top
   d. SST

16. Which activity can contaminate a blood specimen and affect the testing performed on it?
   a. Cleaning the site with alcohol before drawing an ETOH specimen.
   b. Collecting blood cultures before the povidone–iodine is totally dry.
   c. Using povidone–iodine to clean the site prior to a finger puncture.
   d. All of the above activities can affect testing done on the specimen.

17. Which activity is least likely to lead to failure to draw blood?
   a. Choosing a vein that has patency
   b. Leaving the tourniquet on too long
   c. Loosely anchoring the vein
   d. Using a tube that was dropped

18. The best way to keep a vein from rolling is to:
    a. insert the needle at a 45-degree angle.
    b. make certain to anchor it well.
    c. tie the tourniquet very tight.
    d. use a large-diameter needle.

19. You insert the needle in a patient's arm and properly engage the tube. No blood flows into the tube. You make subtle needle adjustments and there is still no blood flow. Which of the following is the best thing to do next?
    a. Discontinue the draw and try somewhere else.
    b. Keep redirecting the needle until you hit a vein.
    c. Lift up on the needle to create a steeper angle.
    d. Try a new tube in case it is a vacuum problem.

20. Which of the following is most likely to affect test results?
    a. Edema
    b. Petechiae
    c. Reflux
    d. Syncope

CASE STUDIES

Case Study 9-1 Problem Sites, Complications, and Procedural Errors

Erica is a recent phlebotomy program graduate who was hired less than a month ago by a major hospital in her first job as a phlebotomist. Her first 3 months of employment are a probationary period, and she is determined to do a good job. This morning she has been asked to collect a stat CBC and electrolytes from a patient in an intensive care unit. The patient is responsive and cooperative but has difficulty breathing. The patient's nurse mentions that she will hook up the patient's oxygen therapy as soon as the phlebotomist is finished with him. He has an IV in his left hand. Erica palpates the right antecubital area. She can feel the median cubital vein but it is deep. The basilic vein is visible and prominent, so she decides to use it to collect the specimen. When she inserts the needle into the arm, the vein rolls and her needle ends up beside the vein and slightly under it. She redirects the needle and the vein rolls again. The patient winces in pain but says nothing. Noticing the look of pain on the patient's face, Erica asks him if it hurts. The patient says yes and tells her that the pain is radiating down his arm and his fingers are tingling. Erica asks him if he would like her to remove the needle. The patient replies "No, you've got to get the specimen," so Erica tries again to redirect the needle. Finally, blood spurts into the tube and a hematoma starts to form quickly. At first Erica thinks that she may have hit an artery, but the specimen is normal in color so Erica dismisses the thought. She quickly collects the specimens, covers the site with gauze and asks the patient to hold pressure while she labels the tubes. When she has finished she thanks the patient and delivers the stat specimens to the laboratory.

QUESTIONS

1. What site selection issues were associated with the collection of this specimen?
2. Were the site selection issues handled properly? Explain why or why not.
3. What complications and procedural errors were involved?
4. Were complications and procedural errors handled properly? Explain why or why not.

IV IS THE FIRST ISSUE, & DEEP MEDIAL CUBITAL

(1) SHE USED THE BASILLIC VEIN SHOULD AND SHOULD OF ATTEMPTED THE MEDIAL CUBITAL VEIN, SHE SHOULD OF TERMINATED THE TEST, SHE SHOULD OF APPLIED PRESSURE AND SHE JUST PUT GAUZE & LEFT.

(2) NO, THE BASILLIC VEIN IS ALWAYS THE 3RD OPTION,

(3) HEMATOMA, SHARP RADING PAIN, TINGLING & DIDN'T WRITE ARTERIAL BLOOD.

(4) NO, FOR COMPLICATIONS THEY WEREN'T MET. BECAUSE SHE DIDN'T APPLY THE PRESSURE AND DIDN'T STOP AFTER THE PAITENT FELT PAIN.

Case Study 9-2 Specimen Quality Concerns

Ray, a newly hired phlebotomist who has just recently finished phlebotomy training, is preparing to draw the last GTT specimen on an outpatient. This is the first GTT he has performed without supervision, and he is proud of how well he has done. The patient has good veins in both arms so he has been alternating arms for the blood draws. The patient is anxious to go home and Ray is in a hurry to go on break, so he quickly selects a vein, performs a successful venipuncture, and collects the required gray-top tube. He finishes the draw and quickly shakes the tube. Later, as he starts to label it, he notices that the tube is only half full. He has been allowed to submit other partial tubes without a problem, so he shrugs his shoulders and proceeds to bandage and then dismiss the patient. He submits the specimen to the lab and goes on break. When he returns he is informed that the last GTT specimen was hemolyzed and unsuitable for testing, so that the test will have to be repeated. Ray is completely surprised by this because there were no problems with the draw. Now Ray has to call the patient and reschedule the test. The patient is understandably upset.

QUESTIONS

1. What errors did Ray make that could have caused hemolysis of the specimen?
2. What could Ray have done differently that might have prevented the hemolysis?
3. What other error did Ray make?
4. What could Ray have done differently to prevent the error in number 3 above?

CHAPTER

10

Capillary Puncture Equipment and Procedures

OBJECTIVES

Study the information in your textbook that corresponds to each objective to prepare yourself for the activities in this chapter.

1. Define the key terms and abbreviations listed at the beginning of this chapter.
2. List and describe the various types of equipment needed for capillary specimen collection.
3. Describe the composition of capillary specimens, identify which tests have different reference values when collected by capillary puncture methods, and name tests that cannot be performed on capillary specimens.
4. Identify indications for performing capillary puncture on adults, children, and infants.
5. List the order of draw for collecting capillary specimens.
6. Describe the proper procedure for selecting the puncture site and collecting capillary specimens from adults, infants, and children.
7. Describe how both routine and thick blood smears are made and the reasons for making them at the collection site.
8. Explain the clinical significance of capillary blood gas, neonatal bilirubin, and newborn screening tests, and describe how specimens for these tests are collected.

Matching

Use choices only once unless otherwise indicated.

MATCHING 10-1: KEY TERMS AND DESCRIPTIONS

Match the key term with the *best* description.

Key Terms (1–10)

1. _____ arterialized
2. _____ blood film/smear
3. _____ calcaneus
4. _____ CBGs
5. _____ cyanotic
6. _____ differential
7. _____ feather
8. _____ galactosemia
9. _____ hypothyroidism
10. _____ interstitial fluid

Descriptions (1–10)

A. A drop of blood spread thin on a microscope slide
B. Bluish in color from lack of oxygen
C. Capillary blood gases; blood gas tests on a capillary specimen
D. Disorder characterized by an inherited inability to metabolize a milk sugar
E. Disorder characterized by insufficient levels of thyroid hormones
F. Fluid in the tissue spaces between the cells
G. Medical term for heel bone
H. Microscopic examination of a blood smear to identify number, type, and characteristics of blood cells
I. Term used to describe a capillary specimen collected from a warmed site
J. Thinnest area of a properly made blood smear where a differential is performed

Key Terms (11–20)

11. _____ intracellular fluid
12. _____ lancet
13. _____ microcollection containers
14. _____ microhematocrit tubes
15. _____ newborn/neonatal screening
16. _____ osteochondritis
17. _____ osteomyelitis
18. _____ PKU
19. _____ posterior curvature
20. _____ whorls

Descriptions (11–20)

A. Back of the heel
B. Disorder involving a defect in the metabolism of phenylalanine
C. Fluid within the cells
D. Inflammation of the bone and cartilage
E. Inflammation of the bone marrow and adjacent bone
F. Narrow-bore 50 to 75 mL capillary tubes
G. Routine testing of newborns for the presence of certain disorders
H. Sharp-pointed or bladed instrument used for capillary puncture
I. Special small plastic tubes used to collect capillary specimens
J. Spiral pattern of the fingerprint

MATCHING 10-2: FINGER PUNCTURE PRECAUTION AND RATIONALE

Match the finger puncture precaution with the appropriate rationale.

Finger Puncture Precaution

1. _____ *Do not* puncture fingers of infants and children under 1 year of age.
2. _____ *Do not* puncture fingers on the same side as a mastectomy without consultation with the patient's physician.

Finger Puncture Rationale

A. Blood can run down the finger rather than form a rounded drop, and make collection difficult.
B. It has a pulse, indicating an artery in the puncture area.
C. The amount of tissue between skin surface and bone is so small that bone injury is very likely.
D. The arm is susceptible to infection, and effects of lymphostasis can lead to erroneous results.

3. _____ *Do not* puncture parallel to the grooves or lines of the fingerprint.
4. _____ *Do not* puncture the fifth or little (pinky) finger.
5. _____ *Do not* puncture the index finger.
6. _____ *Do not* puncture the side or very tip of the finger.
7. _____ *Do not* puncture the thumb.

E. The distance between skin surface and bone is half as much as in the central fleshy portion.
F. The finger is more sensitive and can be more calloused and harder to puncture.
G. Tissue between the skin surface and bone is thinnest in this finger, and bone injury is likely.

MATCHING 10-3: HEEL PUNCTURE PRECAUTION AND RATIONALE

Heel Puncture Precaution

1. _____ *Do not* puncture any deeper than 2.0 mm.
2. _____ *Do not* puncture areas between the imaginary boundaries.
3. _____ *Do not* puncture in the arch and any areas of the foot other than the heel.
4. _____ *Do not* puncture severely bruised areas.
5. _____ *Do not* puncture the posterior curvature of the heel.
6. _____ *Do not* puncture through previous puncture sites.
7. _____ *Do not* puncture a site that is swollen.

Heel Puncture Rationale

A. Arteries, nerves, tendons, and cartilage in these areas can be injured.
B. Deeper punctures risk injuring the bone, even in the safest puncture areas.
C. Excess tissue fluid in the area could contaminate the specimen.
D. It is painful, and impaired circulation or byproducts of healing can negatively affect the specimen.
E. The bone can be as little as 1 mm deep in this area.
F. The calcaneus may be as little as 2.00 mm deep in this area.
G. This can be painful and can spread previously undetected infection.

MATCHING 10-4: BLOOD SMEAR PROBLEM AND PROBABLE CAUSE

Match the blood smear problem with a probable cause (TEXTBOOK Table 10-2). Use choices only once.

Problem

1. __E__ Absence of feather
2. __B__ Holes in smear
3. __H__ Ridges or uneven thickness
4. __G__ Smear is too thick
5. __~~A~~ F__ Smear is too short
6. __D__ Smear is too long
7. __A__ Smear is too thin

8. __C__ Streaks or tails in feathered edge

Probable Cause

~~A.~~ Blood drop too small
~~B.~~ Dirty slide or fat globules in the blood
~~C.~~ Edge of spreader slide dirty or chipped
~~D.~~ Spreader slide angle too shallow
~~E.~~ Spreader slide lifted before smear was completed
~~F.~~ Spreader slide pushed too quickly
~~G.~~ Patient has high red blood cell count
~~H.~~ Too much pressure applied to spreader slide

Labeling Exercises

LABELING EXERCISE 10-1: ADULT HAND

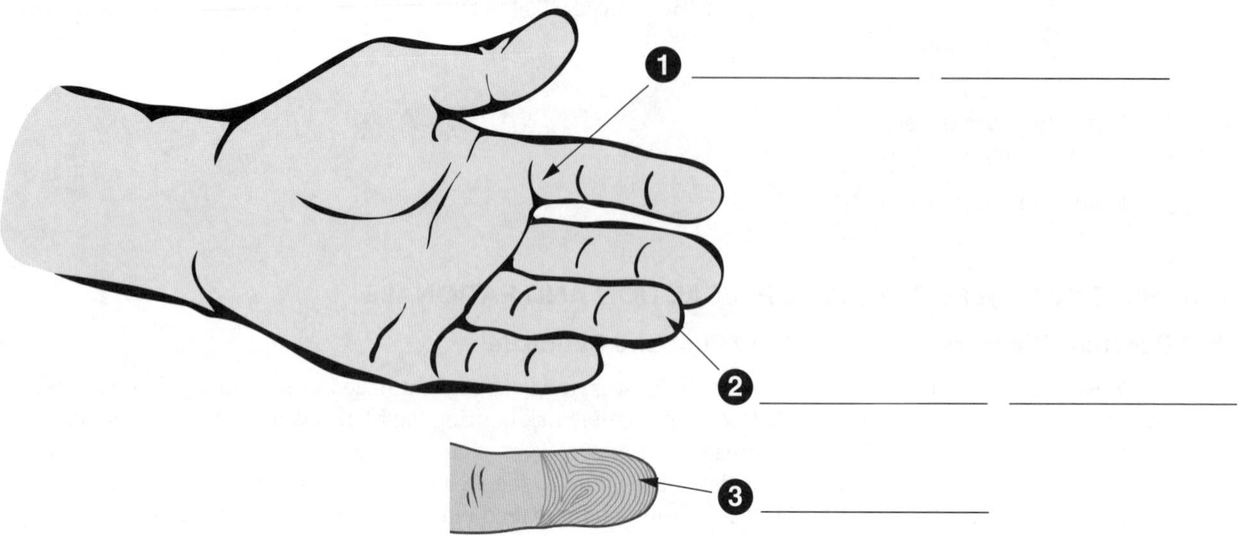

Use directional medical terminology to label the finger parts indicated by arrows 1 and 2. Place an "R" on the fingers that are recommended as capillary puncture sites. Place "NR" on the fingers that are not recommended as capillary puncture sites. Draw a red line to indicate the direction of puncture on an acceptable area of the finger segment identified by arrow number 3. Identify the term for the pattern of the fingerprint shown on the finger segment, and write it on the line after arrow number 3.

LABELING EXERCISE 10-2: INFANT FOOT

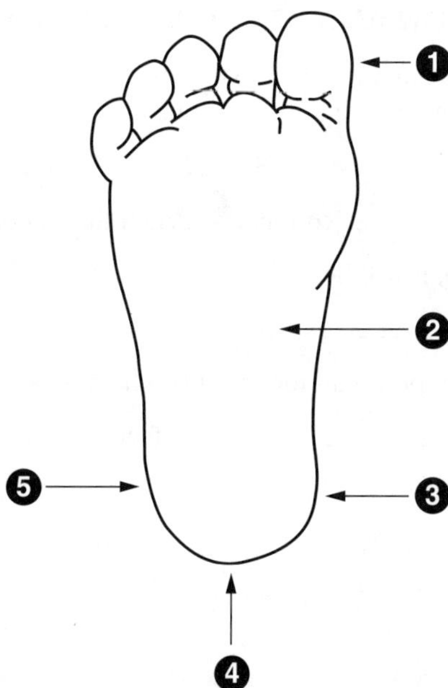

Identify the areas of the infant foot identified by the numbered arrows and write the term for the area on the corresponding numbered line. Use directional medical terms for numbers 3, 4, and 5. In parentheses after each term, write the letter "R" if the site is a recommended heel puncture site and the letters "NR" if it is not a recommended site for heel puncture. Draw dotted lines to indicate the imaginary lines that are used to determine the safe areas for heel puncture. Color the safe areas for heel puncture pink. Draw an "X" in the area of the heel bone and write the medical term for heel bone on line 6 below.

1. ______________________ 4. ______________________

2. ______________________ 5. ______________________

3. ______________________ 6. ______________________

Knowledge Drills

KNOWLEDGE DRILL 10-1: CAUTION AND KEY POINT RECOGNITION

The following sentences are from Caution and Key Point statements found throughout the Chapter 10 text. Using the TEXTBOOK, fill in the blanks with the missing information.

1. Sometimes (A) ____________ blood obtained by (B) ____________ during (C) ________ ______________ situations is put into (D) ________________ containers. When this is done, the specimen must be labeled as (E) ____________ blood. Otherwise, it will be assumed to be a (F) ________________ specimen, which may have different (G) ________________ ____________.
2. Capillary puncture is generally *not* appropriate for patients who are (A) ____________ or have poor (B) ________________ to the (C) ________________ from other causes, such as shock, because (D) ____________ may be hard to obtain and may not be (E) ________________ of (F) ____________ elsewhere in the body.
3. The temperature of the material used to (A) ____________ the (B) ____________ must not exceed (C) ____________ because higher temperatures can (D) ____________the skin, especially the delicate (E) ____________ of an (F) ____________.
4. *Do not* use (A) ____________ to clean skin puncture sites because it greatly interferes with a number of tests, most notably bilirubin, (B) ____________ ____________, (C) ________________, and (D) ________________.
5. Do not squeeze, use strong (A) ________________ pressure, or (B) ____________ the site, as (C) ________________ and (D) ____________ ____________ contamination of the specimen can result.
6. *Do not* use a (A) ________________ motion against the (B) ________________ of the skin and attempt to collect blood as it flows (C) ____________ the (D) ________________. (E) ________________ the (F) ________________ against the skin activates (G) ________________ causing them to (H) ____________, and can also (I) ________________ the specimen.
7. *Do not* apply (A) ________________ to infants and children under (B) ________ years of age because they pose a (C) ____________ hazard. In addition, bandage (D) ____________ can (E) ____________ to the paper-thin skin of newborns and (F) ____________ it when the (G) ________________ is removed.
8. The (A) ____________ ____________ must be (B) ____________ ____________ when collecting a bilirubin specimen to prevent it from (C) ____________ ____________ (D) ________________ in the (E) ________________ as it is collected.
9. If an infant requires a (A) ____________ ________________, newborn screening samples should be collected (B) ____________ it is started, as (C) ________________ of the sample with donor (D) ____________ invalidates test results.
10. Do not contaminate the filter paper (A) ____________ by touching them with or without (B) ____________ or allowing any other object or substance to touch them before, during, or (C) ____________ specimen collection. Substances that have been identified as (D) ________________ in newborn screening specimens include (E) ____________, formula, lotion, powder, and (F) ____________.
11. Blood (A) ____________ are considered (B) ________________ or (C) ________________ until they are (D) ____________ or fixed.

12. Capillary specimen collection is especially useful for (A) ______________ patients in whom removal of (B) ______________ quantities of blood can have (C) ______________ ______________.
13. An important (A) ___________ required lancet safety feature is a permanently (B) ___________ blade or (C) ___________ ___________ to reduce the risk of accidental sharps injury.
14. Although (A) ___________ ___________ top microtubes are available from some manufacturers, they are not to be used for (B) ______________ specimens. They are intended to be used for (C) ___________ ___________ collected by (D) ___________ in difficult draw situations.
15. Pay strict attention to (A) ________ (B) ___________ of microtubes containing (C) ______________.

KNOWLEDGE DRILL 10-2: SCRAMBLED WORDS

1. zalitraerdie ________________________ (blood from a warmed site)
2. liribunbi ________________________ (it can cross the blood–brain barrier)
3. slacneuca ________________________ (do not puncture this)
4. placryail ________________________ (this bed is in the skin)
5. snatrelititi ________________________ (pertaining to spaces between tissue cells)
6. cletan ________________________ (a very sharp object)
7. napartl ________________________ (pertaining to the sole of the foot)
8. pocos ________________________ (not good technique to do this)
9. tairoluvtel ________________________ (light that breaks down bilirubin)
10. slowhr ________________________ (fingerprint pattern)

Skills Drills

SKILLS DRILL 10-1: REQUISITION ACTIVITY

You have received the following test order with instructions to collect the specimens by capillary puncture. List (according to the order of draw) the name of the test that will be collected in each tube, the stopper colors of the microtubes you will use, the additive(s) the tubes contain, and any special handling required for each specimen. Write "NA" if no special handling is required.

Any Hospital USA
1123 West Physician Drive
Any Town USA

Laboratory Test Requisition

PATIENT INFORMATION:

Name: Smith (last) John (first) L (MI)

Identification Number: 051263975 Birth Date: ________

Referring Physician: Payne

Date to be Collected: 05/12/2011 Time to be Collected: STAT

Special Instructions: Collect by capillary puncture only

TEST(S) REQUIRED:

____ NH4 – Ammonia	____ Gluc – glucose
X Bili – Bilirubin, total & direct	____ Hgb – hemoglobin
____ BMP – basic metabolic panel	____ Lact – lactic acid/lactate
____ BUN - Blood urea nitrogen	____ Plt. Ct. – platelet count
X Lytes – electrolytes	____ PT – prothrombin time
X CBC – complete blood count	____ PTT – partial thromboplastin time
____ Chol – cholesterol	____ RPR – rapid plasma reagin
____ ESR – erythrocyte sed rate	____ T&S – type and screen
____ EtOH - alcohol	____ PSA – prostate specific antigen
____ D-dime	

Test in Order of Draw	Stopper Color	Tube Additive	Special Handling
1. CBC	LAVENDER	EDTA	
2. LYTES	GREEN	HEPARIN	
3. BILI	GREEN	↓	COVER IT FROM LIGHT

SKILLS DRILL 10-2: WORD BUILDING

Divide each of the words below into all of its elements (parts); prefix (P), word root (WR), combining vowel (CV), and suffix (S). Write the word part, its definition, and the meaning of the word on the corresponding lines. If the word does not have a particular element, write "NA" (not applicable) in its place. (See Chapter 4 of the TEXTBOOK.)

Example: pathologist

Elements *NA* / *path* / *o* / *logist*
P WR CV S

Definitions *NA* / *disease* / *NA* / *specialist in the study of*

Meaning: a specialist who studies and interprets disease

1. osteochondritis

Elements ______ / ______ / ____ / ______ / ______
P WR CV WR S

Definitions ______ / ______ / ____ / ______

Meaning:

2. microhematocrit

Elements ______ / ______ / ____ / ______
P WR CV S

Definitions ______ / ______ / ____ / ______

Meaning:

3. hemolyze

Elements ______ / ______ / ____ / ______
P WR CV S

Definitions ______ / ______ / ____ / ______

Meaning:

4. hypothyroidism

Elements ______ / ______ / ____ / ______
P WR CV S

Definitions ______ / ______ / ____ / ______

Meaning:

5. dermal

Elements ______ / ______ / ____ / ______
P WR CV S

Definitions ______ / ______ / ____ / ______

Meaning:

6. cyanotic

Elements ______ / ______ / ____ / ______
P WR CV S

Definitions ______ / ______ / ____ / ______

Meaning:

SKILLS DRILL 10-3: FINGERSTICK PROCEDURE (Textbook Procedure 10-1)

Fill in the blanks with the missing information.

Steps	Explanation/Rationale
1–3. See Chapter 8 Venipuncture steps 1 through 3.	See Chapter 8 Procedure 8-2: steps 1 through 3.
4. (1) __________ hands and put on (2) __________.	Proper hand hygiene plays a major role in (3) __________ __________ by protecting the phlebotomist, the patient, and others from contamination. Gloves are required at this point to protect the phlebotomist from bloodborne pathogen exposure.
5. Position the patient.	The patient's arm must be supported on a (4) __________ surface with the hand extended and the palm up. A young child may have to be held on the lap and restrained by a parent or guardian.
6. Select the puncture/incision site.	Select a site in the central, (5) __________ portion and slightly to the side of center of a (6) __________ or (7) __________ finger that is warm, pink or normal color, and free of scars, cuts, bruises, infection, rashes, swelling, or (8) __________ punctures.
7. (9) __________ the site, if applicable.	Warming makes blood collection easier and (10) __________, and reduces the tendency to squeeze the site. It is not normally part of a routine fingerstick unless the hand is cold; in which case, wrap it in a comfortably warm washcloth or towel for 3 to 5 minutes or use a commercial (11) __________ __________.
8. Clean and (12) __________ __________ the site.	CLSI recommends (13) __________ __________ for cleaning capillary puncture sites. Cleaning removes or inhibits skin flora that could infiltrate the puncture and cause infection. Letting the site dry naturally permits maximum (14) __________, action, prevents contamination caused by wiping, and avoids stinging on puncture and specimen hemolysis from residual alcohol.

9. Prepare the equipment.	Select a fingerstick (15) ___________ according to the age of the patient and amount of blood to be collected. Verify lancet (16) ___________ by checking to see that packaging is intact before opening; open and handle aseptically to maintain sterility. Select collection devices according to the ordered tests. Place items within easy reach along with several layers of gauze or gauze-type pads. Remove or release any lancet (17) ___________ mechanism and hold the lancet between the thumb and index finger, or per manufacturer's instructions.
10. Puncture the site and (18) ___________ the lancet/incision device.	Grasp the patient's finger between your nondominant (19) ___________ and ___________ finger, holding it securely in case of sudden movement. Place the lancet (20) ___________ against the skin in the central, fleshy pad of the finger, slightly to the side of center to avoid bone injury, and (21) ___________ to the fingerprint whorls so the blood will form easily collected drops and not run down the fingerprint. Warn the patient or parent/guardian, trigger the puncture, and discard the lancet in sharps container.
11. Wipe away the (22) ___________ blood drop.	Apply gentle pressure until a (23) ___________ ___________ forms, and use a clean gauze pad to wipe it away. This prevents contamination of the specimen with excess (24) ___________ ___________ and rids the site of alcohol residue that could prevent formation of well-rounded drops and also hemolyze the specimen.
12. Fill and mix the tubes/containers in (25) ___________ ___________ ___________.	Collect subsequent blood drops using devices appropriate for the ordered tests and in the CLSI order of draw to (26) ___________ effects of clotting on specimens. Hold a microhematocrit tube above or beside the site and touch one end to the (27) ___________ ___________. You may need to lower the opposite end of the tube slightly as it fills, but do not remove it from the drop because this creates air spaces in the specimen that compromise

results. When the tube is full, (28) __________ the opposite or dry end with (29) __________ or other suitable sealant. Hold a microcollection tube below the blood drop. Touch the scoop to the blood drop and allow it to (30) __________ __________ the inside wall of the tube. The tube may need a gentle (31) __________ occasionally to settle blood to the bottom. Seal tubes when full and mix additive tubes by gently inverting them (32) __________ to __________ times.

13. Place gauze and apply (33) __________.

Apply pressure with a clean gauze pad and elevate the site until bleeding stops.

14. (34) __________ the specimen and observe special handling instructions.

Specimens must be labeled with the appropriate information (see Chapter 8). Affix labels (35) __________ to microcollection containers. Place microhematocrit tubes in a nonadditive or aliquot tube and place the label on this container. Follow any special handling required.

15. (36) __________ the site and apply bandage.

Examine the site to verify that bleeding has stopped; apply a bandage if the patient is an older child or adult, and advise the patient to keep it in place for at least (37) __________ __________. If bleeding persists beyond (38) __________ __________ notify the patient's nurse or physician.

16. Dispose of used and (39) __________ materials.

Discard equipment packaging and bandage wrappers in the trash. Follow (40) __________ protocol for discarding contaminated items, such as (41) __________-__________ gauze.

17. Thank patient, remove gloves, and (42) __________ hands.

Thanking the patient is courteous and professional. Remove gloves (43) __________ and wash or decontaminate hands with (44) __________ as an infection control precaution.

18. Transport specimen to the lab.

(45) __________ delivery to the lab is necessary to protect specimen integrity.

SKILLS DRILL 10-4: HEELSTICK PROCEDURE RATIONALE (Text Procedure 10-2)

Match the following rationales to the heelstick procedure steps listed below. Place the appropriate letter next to the step under Rationale.

A. Removes or inhibits skin flora that could infiltrate the puncture and cause infection
B. The infant should be lying face up with foot lower than the torso so gravity can assist blood flow
C. Open and handle aseptically to maintain sterility
D. Request is reviewed for completeness, date and time of collection, status, and priority
E Makes blood collection easier and faster
F. Follow CLSI order of draw for capillary specimens to minimize effects of clotting
G. Correct ID is vital to patient safety and meaningful test results
H. Place the lancet flat against the skin using enough pressure to keep it in place without deeply compressing the skin
I. Exposure to latex can trigger a life-threatening reaction in those allergic to it
J. Prevents contamination of the specimen with excess tissue fluid
K. Medial or lateral plantar surface of the heel that is warm and normal color
L. Applying pressure and elevating the foot helps stop bleeding
M. Proper hand hygiene plays a major role in infection control by protecting the phlebotomist, the patient, and others from contamination

Heelstick Procedure Step	Rationale
1. Review and accession test request.	______
2. Approach, identify, and prepare patient.	______
3. Verify diet restrictions and latex sensitivity.	______
4. Sanitize hands and put on gloves.	______
5. Position the patient.	______
6. Select the puncture site.	______
7. Warm the site, if applicable.	______
8. Clean and air-dry the site.	______
9. Prepare the equipment.	______
10. Puncture the site and discard the lancet/incision device.	______
11. Wipe away the first blood drop.	______
12. Fill and mix tubes/containers in order of draw.	______
13. Place gauze and apply pressure.	______

SKILLS DRILL 10-5: BLOOD SPOT COLLECTION PROCEDURE HIGHLIGHTS (Textbook Procedure 10-4)

The following are highlights from the newborn screening blood spot collection procedure. Fill in the blanks with the missing information.

1. Bring the filter paper close to the heel: The (A) ____________ must not actually (B) ____________ the (C) ____________; if it does, (D) ____________, incomplete (E) ____________ of the paper, (F) ____________, and stoppage of (G) ____________ can result.
2. Generate a large, free-flowing drop of blood: Small drops can result in incomplete (A) ____________ and the tendency to (B) ____________ successive drops in a circle to (C) ____________ it.
3. Touch the blood drop to the center of the filter paper circle: The drop must touch the center of the circle for (A) ____________ to (B) ____________ (C) ____________ out to the (D) ____________.
4. Fill the circle with blood: Blood drop position is (A) ____________ until blood (B) ____________ through the circle, completely filling (C) ____________ ____________ of the paper. Caution: Do not fill spots from the (D) ____________ to finish filling the circles because this causes (E) ____________ and (F) ____________ results.
5. Fill remaining blood spot circles: Fill (A) ________ circles the same way. (B) ____________ or (C) ____________ filled circles can result in (D) ____________ to perform all required (E) ________.
6. Check the site: Check the site to verify that bleeding has (A) ____________, but do not apply a (B) ____________ because it can become a (C) ____________ hazard and can also (D) ____________ the skin when removed.
7. Allow the specimen to air-dry: The specimen must be allowed to air-dry in an elevated (A) ____________ position away from heat or (B) ____________. It should not be (C) ____________ to dry or (D) ____________ with other specimens before, during, or after the drying process. (E) ____________ causes blood to (F) ____________ to the (G) ________ ________ of the filter paper and leads to erroneous test results.

Crossword

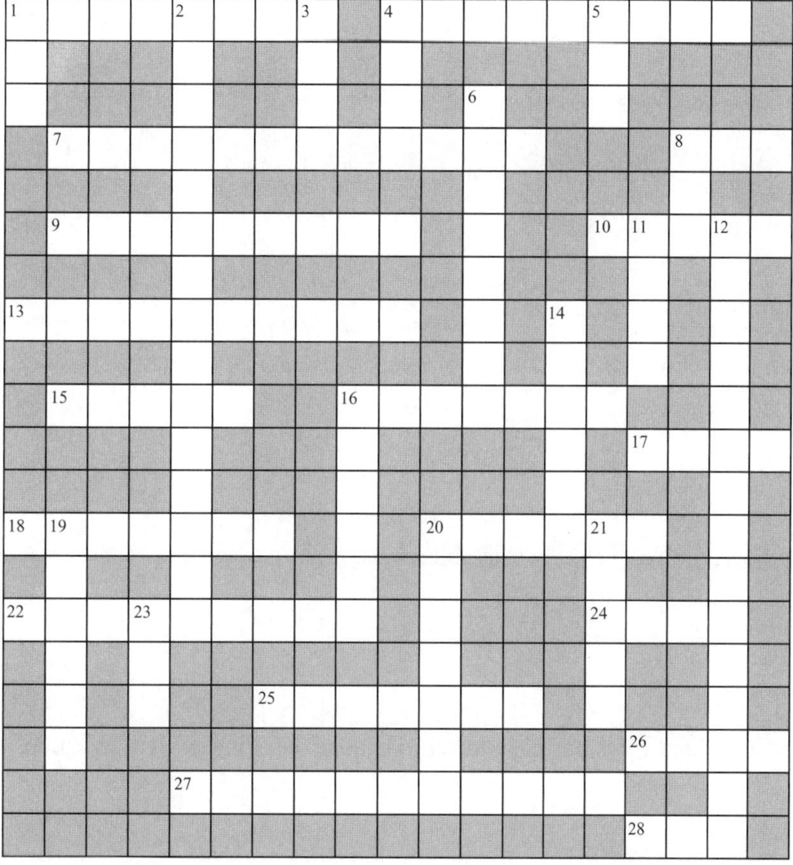

ACROSS

1. Marked by bluish color
4. Blood specimen type collected by a dermal puncture
7. Capillary blood becomes this after warming the site
8. Alcohol ____ used for cleaning the site
9. Heel bone
10. Digit not suggested for capillary collection
13. Small plastic tubes used to collect tiny amounts of blood
15. Rectangular glass plate required for making a blood smear
16. Clay for plugging microhematocrit tube
17. Testing done at the location of the patient (abbrev.)
18. Bottom surface of the foot
20. Spiral pattern of the fingerprint
22. Cuts in the skin
24. Place chosen to collect blood sample
25. Neonatal
26. Outer covering of the body
27. Contaminating factor when doing capillary collections (2 words)
28. Hemolysis in newborns (abbrev.)

DOWN

1. Capillary blood gas (abbrev.)
2. Inflammation of the bone and cartilage
3. Regulations that establish standards for all laboratory facilities
4. Organization that offers phlebotomy standards
5. Leukocyte alkaline phosphatase
6. Pertaining to newborn
8. Genetic disorder associated with phenylalanine
11. Recommended collection site for infants
12. Term for obtaining tiny amounts of blood by capillary puncture
14. Recommended site for capillary puncture on children over 1 year of age
16. Container for used lancets and needles
19. Sterile, disposable, bladed instrument
20. Necessary to ____ ____ first drop of blood
21. Perforates the skin without a lancet
23. Units in the nursery where severely ill newborns can be monitored

Chapter Review Questions

1. An inherited metabolic disorder detected through newborn screening.
   a. Diabetes
   b. Glucose
   c. Phenylketonuria
   d. Potassium

2. Which of the following equipment is needed for a malaria test?
   a. Capillary tube
   b. Clay sealant
   c. Glass slide
   d. Microhematocrit tube

3. A plasma specimen for this type of test cannot be collected by capillary puncture.
   a. Chemistry
   b. Coagulation
   c. Hematology
   d. All of the above

4. Capillary blood composition more closely resembles:
   a. arterial blood.
   b. lymph fluid.
   c. tissue fluid.
   d. venous blood.

5. The concentration of this analyte is normally lower in capillary specimens than in venous specimens:
   a. calcium.
   b. glucose.
   c. hemoglobin.
   d. all of the above.

6. Capillary collection is the preferred method of blood collection in infants because:
   a. an infant can be injured by the restraining method used.
   b. removing larger quantities of blood can lead to anemia.
   c. venipuncture may damage veins and surrounding tissue.
   d. all of the above.

7. If using capillary puncture to collect the following microtubes from a patient, which one would be collected first?
   a. Gray top
   b. Green top
   c. Purple top
   d. Red top

8. Which of the following is a recommended site for finger puncture in adults?
   a. End segment of the little finger
   b. Distal segment of the middle finger
   c. Plantar surface of the index finger
   d. Proximal segment of the ring finger

9. The medial plantar surface of the heel is located
   a. at the very back portion of the heel.
   b. in the middle of the bottom of the heel.
   c. on the big toe side of the bottom of the heel.
   d. on the little toe side of the bottom of the heel.

10. It is necessary to control the depth of lancet insertion during heel puncture to avoid
    a. bacterial contamination.
    b. bone injury.
    c. excessive bleeding.
    d. puncturing a vein.

11. The primary purpose of warming a capillary puncture site is to
    a. delay clotting.
    b. increase blood flow.
    c. minimize contamination.
    d. reduce hemoconcentration.

12. Skin pain fibers increase in abundance
    a. in the upper epidermis.
    b. below 2.4 mm in depth.
    c. beyond 4.9 mm in depth.
    d. within the vascular bed.

13. Adult capillary puncture may be performed when
    a. there are no accessible veins.
    b. the patient has thrombotic tendencies.
    c. veins must be saved for chemotherapy.
    d. all of the above.

14. Wipe away the first drop of blood during capillary puncture to
    a. minimize tissue fluid contamination
    b. reduce the chance of hemolysis.
    c. remove any alcohol residue.
    d. all of the above.

15. Do *not* use povidone–iodine to clean skin puncture sites because it interferes with
    a. potassium results.
    b. phosphorus results.
    c. uric acid results.
    d. all of the above.

16. Which of the following represents proper capillary specimen collection technique?
    a. Clean the site with alcohol and wipe it dry so it will not sting.
    b. Puncture the skin parallel to the whorls of the fingerprint.
    c. Squeeze the finger hard to get the very best blood flow.
    d. Touch the scoop to the blood drop, not the skin surface.

17. Blood smears made using EDTA specimens should be prepared within:
    a. 1 hour of specimen collection.
    b. 2 hours of specimen collection.
    c. 6 hours of specimen collection.
    d. 24 hours of specimen collection.

18. An infant bilirubin specimen is collected in an amber microtube to:
    a. flag it as a capillary specimen.
    b. identify it as a bilirubin specimen.
    c. protect the specimen from light.
    d. reduce the chance of hemolysis.

19. Which of the following PKU collection techniques is incorrect?
    a. Air-dry the slips horizontally.
    b. Completely fill every circle.
    c. Do not touch the filter paper.
    d. Fill circles from both sides.

20. Which of the following can result in a blood smear that is too long?
    a. Angle of spreader slide is too steep.
    b. Blood drop is too large or too thin.
    c. Spreader slide is pushed too quickly.
    d. Patient has a high hemoglobin level.

CASE STUDIES

Case Study 10-1 Neonatal Bilirubin Collection

A newly OJT (on the job) trained phlebotomist was sent to the newborn nursery to collect a bilirubin specimen. This was the first time she had collected an infant specimen by herself, and she was anxious to do a good job. The infant was under a UV light, and, although she thought it should be turned off, both nurses in the room were busy with a procedure on another infant and she didn't want to interrupt them to ask permission, so she decided to obtain the specimen quickly without turning it off. She rapidly cleaned the site and made the puncture. The blood came slowly and it took her awhile to collect the specimen. She finally filled an amber bullet to an acceptable level, labeled it, put an adhesive bandage on the infant's heel, and delivered the specimen to the lab.

QUESTIONS

1. Why was the infant placed under a UV light?
2. Should the light have been turned off during specimen collection? Why or why not?
3. What might be the consequences of leaving the UV light on during specimen collection?
4. What could the phlebotomist have done to make the collection go more quickly?
5. What other error did the phlebotomist make that could have caused injury to the infant after she left the nursery?

Case Study 10-2 Capillary Specimen Collection Technique and Order of Draw

A phlebotomist had a request to collect STAT electrolytes on a patient and a CBC that was not STAT. The patient had an IV just above the wrist in the left arm. The right antecubital area was badly bruised, and the patient did not have any suitable veins in either hand. Consequently, the phlebotomist decided to collect the specimens by capillary puncture, choosing the right middle finger as the collection site. After making the puncture, the phlebotomist decided to collect the electrolytes first because they were STAT and he was having a difficult time getting good blood flow. He was able to fill the green top bullet for the electrolytes and proceeded to collect the CBC. He had to use a lot of pressure on the finger to keep the blood flowing, but he eventually filled a lavender bullet for the CBC to a proper level. After the samples had been submitted to the lab he was told to recollect the CBC because the results were questionable.

QUESTIONS

1. What was most likely wrong with the CBC results?
2. Why was only the CBC affected?
3. What could the phlebotomist have done differently to protect the CBC?
4. What should the phlebotomist do differently when he recollects the specimen?

UNIT III CROSSWORD EXERCISE

ACROSS

1. Antiseptics inhibit their growth
4. Spiral pattern that forms the fingerprint
6. Blood gas performed on ND (abbrev.)
8. Eutectic mixture of local anesthetics
9. Term used to describe milky white or turbid serum or plasma
11. Intravenous (abbrev.)
12. Anticoagulant typically used for hematology studies
13. Holding a vein in place by pulling the skin taut
15. Preanalytical errors can affect ________ results
16. Metabolism of glucose by blood cells
18. Record in the order received
20. ETS additive for blood culture specimens
22. Number that relates to the diameter of the needle lumen
23. Anticoagulant in tubes with light blue tops
25. Atrioventricular valve (abbrev.)
26. Property of thixotropic gel that changes during centrifugation
29. Pertaining to veins
30. Central venous access device
33. Excessive and persistent fear
37. Medical term for fainting
38. Examine by touch or feel

DOWN

1. Winged infusion set
2. Anticoagulants prevent it
3. Backflow of blood from an evacuated tube into a patient's vein
4. Do this to the site to arterialize a specimen
5. Internal space of a vessel or tube
7. Later product of red blood cell breakdown
10. Tiny red spots that appear on the skin upon tourniquet application
13. Substance that keeps blood from clotting
14. Destruction of RBCs and release of hemoglobin into the fluid of a specimen
17. Hardened
18. Prefix meaning against
19. Immediately
21. Container used to dispose of used needles and lancets
24. Condition characterized by high bilirubin levels
27. Combining form meaning bone
28. Fossa on ventral side of the arm (abbrev.)
31. Type of blood sampling device
32. Bedside or alternate site testing (abbrev.)
34. NB screening test for an amino acid metabolic disorder (abbrev.)
35. Written and signed order not to resuscitate (abbrev.)
36. Glass tube top color indicating no additive

CHAPTER 11

Special Collections and Point-of-Care Testing

OBJECTIVES

Study the information in your textbook that corresponds to each objective to prepare yourself for the activities in this chapter.

1. Define the key terms and abbreviations at the beginning of this chapter.
2. Explain the principle behind each special collection procedure, identify the steps involved, and list any special supplies or equipment required.
3. Describe patient identification and specimen labeling procedures required for blood bank tests and identify the types of specimens typically required.
4. Describe sterile technique in blood culture collection, explain why it is important, and list the reasons why a physician might order blood cultures.
5. List examples of coagulation specimens and describe how to properly collect and handle them.
6. Describe chain-of-custody procedures and identify the tests that may require them.
7. Explain the importance of timing; identify the role of drug half-life, providing names of drugs as examples; and describe peak, trough, and therapeutic levels in therapeutic drug monitoring.
8. Define point-of-care testing (POCT), explain the principle behind the POCT examples listed in this chapter, and identify any special equipment required.

Matching

Use choices only once unless otherwise indicated.

MATCHING 11-1: KEY TERMS AND DESCRIPTIONS

Match the key term with the *best* description.

Key Terms (1–18)

1. ______ ACT
2. ______ Aerobic
3. ______ Anaerobic
4. ______ ARD
5. ______ autologous
6. ______ BAC
7. ______ Bacteremia
8. ______ BNP
9. ______ BT
10. ______ Chain of custody
11. ______ Compatibility
12. ______ CRP
13. ______ EQC
14. ______ ETOH
15. ______ FAN
16. ______ FUO
17. ______ GTT
18. ______ HCG

Descriptions (1–18)

A. Abbreviation for ethanol
B. Activated clotting time
C. Antimicrobial removal device
D. Bacteria in the blood
E. Platelet function test
F. Instrument's electronic QC check
G. Donating blood for one's own use.
H. Without air or able to live without oxygen
I. Fastidious antimicrobial neutralization
J. Fever of unknown origin
K. Cardiac hormone produced in response to pressure overload
L. Hormone detected with POCT pregnancy test
M. Detailed documentation for forensic specimens collections
N. Ability to be mixed together without unfavorable effects
O. Test used to diagnose carbohydrate metabolism problems
P. Blood alcohol concentration
Q. With air or able to live only in the presence of oxygen
R. Nonspecific marker for inflammation

Key Terms (19–37)

19. ______ Hypoglycemia
20. ______ Hyperkalemia
21. ______ Hypernatremia
22. ______ iCa^{2+}
23. ______ INR
24. ______ K^+
25. ______ Lactate
26. ______ Lookback
27. ______ Lysis
28. ______ NIDA
29. ______ Peak level
30. ______ POCT

Descriptions (19–37)

A. After a meal
B. Highest serum drug concentration anticipated
C. The mineral potassium
D. Decreased blood sugar levels
E. Drug level testing collected at specific times
F. Specific heart muscle protein staying elevated up to 14 days
G. Standardized form of PT results
H. Ionized form of calcium
I. Microorganism and toxins in the blood
J. National Institute on Drug Abuse
K. Lowest serum drug concentration expected
L. Requires blood unit components to be traceable to the donor
M. Specific heart muscle protein showing elevation in 3 to 6 hours
N. Increased blood sodium levels
O. Rupturing, as in the bursting of a red blood cell
P. Level of this analyte marks severity of metabolic acidosis

31. _____ PP
32. _____ Septicemia
33. _____ TDM
34. _____ TGC
35. _____ TnI
36. _____ TnT
37. _____ Trough level

Q. Testing performed at the patient's side
R. Increased blood potassium
S. Intensive insulin therapy to control glucose levels

MATCHING 11-2: POC TESTS AND INSTRUMENTS USED FOR TESTING

Match the following tests to the POCT instruments (instruments can only be used once).

POC Tests

A. CK-MB
B. Lactate
C. Glycosylated hgb
D. Hemoglobin
E. Pco_2
F. PT
G. TnT
H. BUN
I. BNP
J. Hematocrit
K. β-ketone
L. UA
M. Guaiac
N. HCG
O. CRP
P. Platelet function

POCT Instruments

1. _____ Verify Now
2. _____ Quidel Quick Vue
3. _____ Precision XceedPro
4. _____ StatSpin CritSpin
5. _____ Hemoccult II Sensa
6. _____ CARDIAC T Rapid Assay
7. _____ Cholestech LDX
8. _____ Triage MeterPro
9. _____ GEM Premier 4000
10. _____ HemoCue HB 201+
11. _____ DCA Vantage
12. _____ Triage Cardiac Panel
13. _____ CoaguChek
14. _____ i-STAT
15. _____ ABL80
16. _____ Clinitek 2001

MATCHING 11-3: SPECIAL TEST COLLECTION, EQUIPMENT, OR PROCEDURE

Match the following tests with the special equipment or procedure involved. (Answers can be used only once.)

Special Test

1. _____ 2-hour PP
2. _____ Blood alcohol
3. _____ Blood culture
4. _____ Blood type and screen
5. _____ BT

Special Handling, Equipment, or Procedure

A. Draw in trace element–free tube.
B. Involves intradermal injection of diluted antigen.
C. May require a proctor present at the time of collection.
D. May require photo identification before collection.
E. Requires serial collection of blood specimens at specific times.
F. Patient ID procedures are extra strict.
G. Requires a 9-to-1 ratio of blood to anticoagulant in the collection tube.

6. ______ GTT
7. ______ Paternity testing
8. ______ Polycythemia
9. ______ PT
10. ______ TB test
11. ______ Urine drug screen
12. ______ Zinc

H. Skin antisepsis is critical to accurate test results.
I. Special chain of custody protocol required.
J. Specimen is collected at specific time after eating.
K. Treatment often involves removal of units of blood.
L. Use of a blood pressure cuff is required to perform the test.

Labeling Exercises

LABELING EXERCISE 11-1: POC INSTRUMENTS AND TESTS

Label the photo of each of the following POC instruments with the name of the instrument and the test that it is used to measure. Choose from the following list of tests.

Instrument That Can Measure

Lactate
Hematocrit
Platelet function
ACT
BNP
β-ketones
HCG
HDL
Creatinine
Blood gases

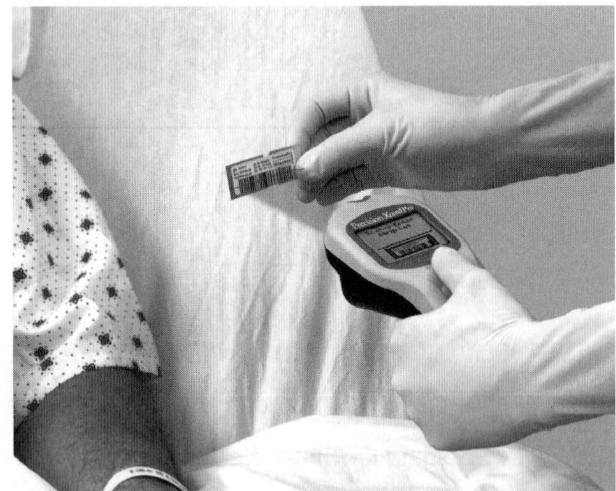

1. name: ________________________ test: ________________________

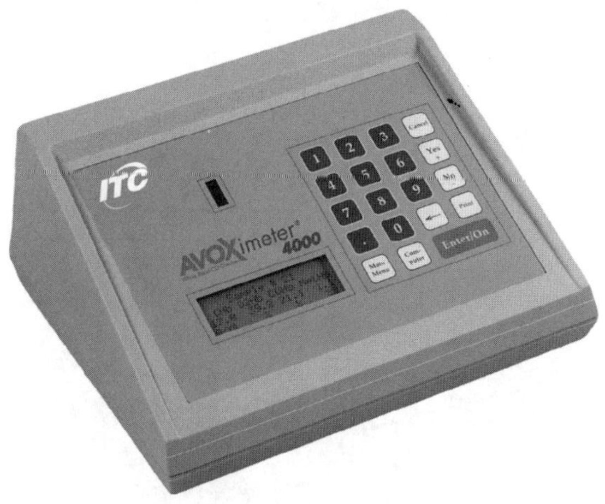

2. name: ______________________ test: ______________________

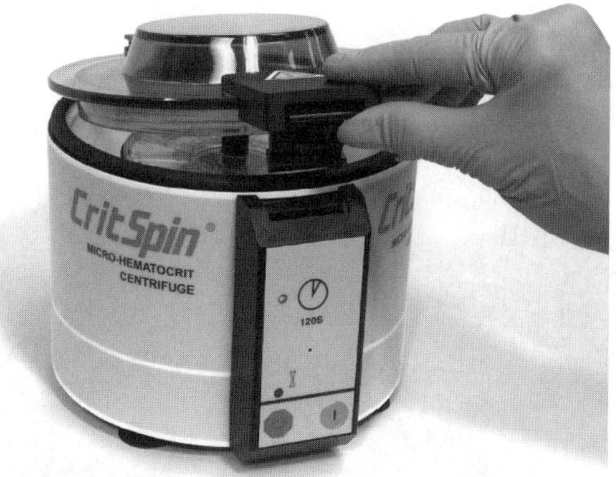

3. name: ______________________ test: ______________________

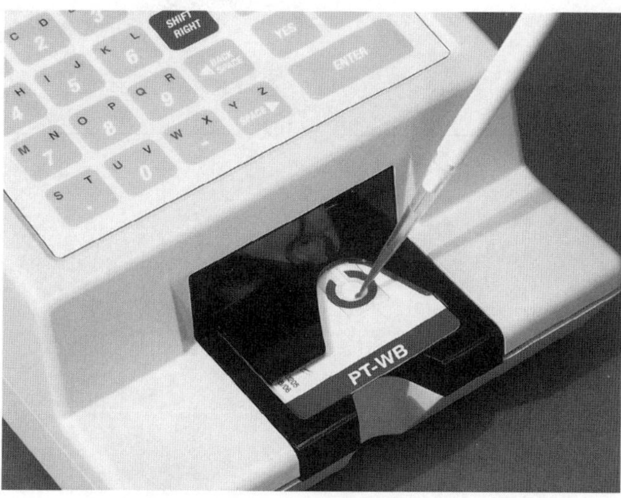

4. name: ______________________ test: ______________________

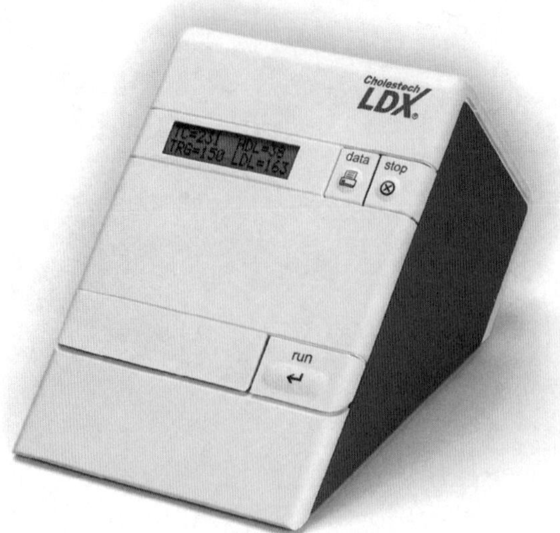

5. name: ______________________ test: ______________________

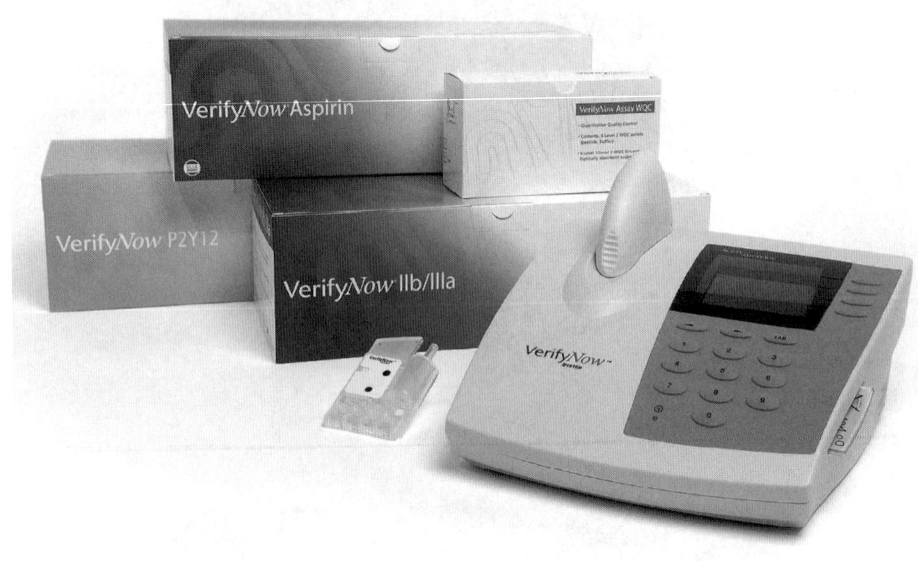

6. name: ______________________ test: ______________________

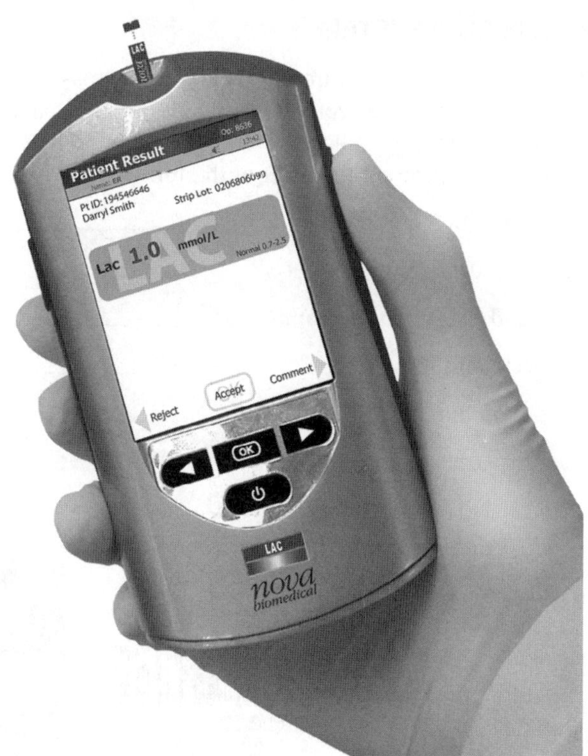

7. name: ______________________ test: ______________________

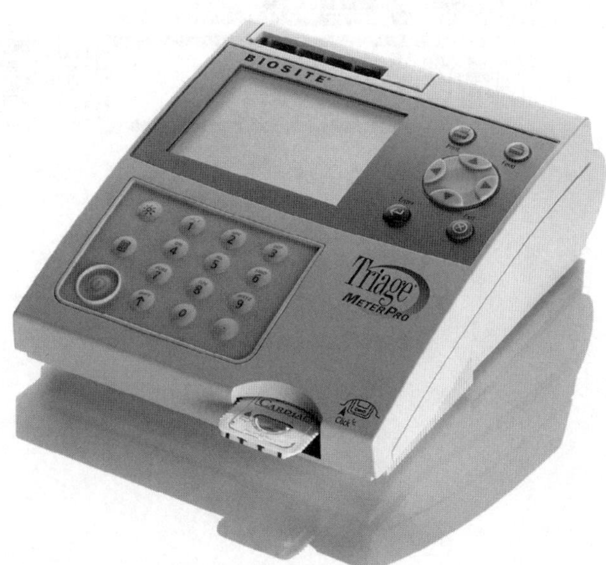

8. name: ______________________ test: ______________________

LABELING EXERCISE 11-2: ONE BBID SYSTEM

You are a new phlebotomist who is asked to get blood from a patient for a cross match STAT. Before leaving the lab with the requisition, the MT in the blood bank gives you a FlexiBlood form and band to use in collecting the specimen. When you get to the floor, you realize that you have several questions on how to use this form. Fortunately, adequate instructions for you to follow are given on the front of the form.

1. Which of the following is the unique BBID number? ____________________
2. Where does the preprinted patient information go? ____________________
3. Which part is filled in, removed, and placed on the band? ____________________
4. Which one is the label for the specimen tube? ____________________
5. What bar-code labels are to be put on the units in the lab? ____________________

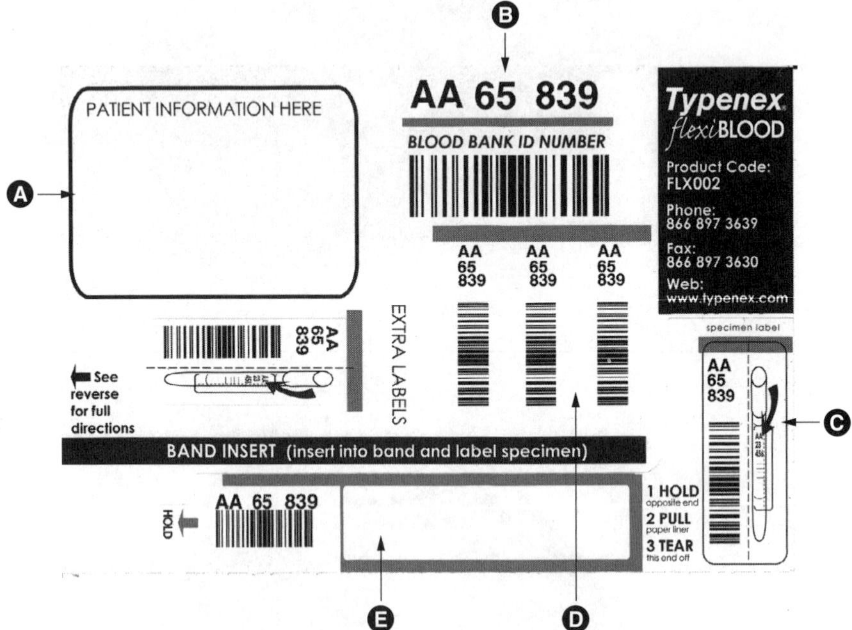

Knowledge Drills

KNOWLEDGE DRILL 11-1: CAUTION AND KEY POINT RECOGNITION

Instructions: The following sentences are taken from caution and key point statements found throughout the chapter. Using the TEXTBOOK, fill in the blanks with the missing information.

1. Blood cultures are typically ordered immediately (A) ____________ or (B) ____________ anticipated (C) ____________ spikes when bacteria are most likely to be present. (D) ____________ collection is essential. Recent studies have shown that the best chance for detecting (E) ____________ exists between (F)____________ minutes to (G) ____________ hours prior to the fever (H) ____________ before the body eliminates some of the microorganisms.
2. According to (A) ____________, the volume of blood drawn for (B) ____________ and younger children should be from (C) ____________ to (D) ____________ of the patient's total (E) ____________ ____________, generally speaking.
3. According to the CLSI, (A) ____________ ____________ is the recommended blood culture site disinfectant for (B) ____________ 2 months and older and patients with (C) ____________ sensitivity.
4. Blood culture specimens are always collected (A) ____________ in the order of draw to prevent (B) ____________ from other tubes.
5. The practice of changing (A) ____________ prior to this transfer is no longer (B) ____________. Several recent studies have shown that (C) ____________ needles has little (D) ____________ on reducing (E) ____________ rates and may actually (F) ____________ risk of (G) ____________ injury to the phlebotomist.
6. If the patient (A) ____________ during the GTT procedure, his or her (B) ____________ must be consulted to determine if the test should be (C) ____________.
7. (A) ____________ tubes are preferred for blood alcohol specimens because of the (B) ____________ nature of (C) ____________ tubes.
8. Regulatory (A) ____________ and the (B) ____________ recommend that a person receive (C) ____________ authorization to perform (D) ____________ glucose testing only after completing (E) ____________ training in facility-established procedures, including (F) ____________ and (G) ____________.
9. (A) ____________ should be repeated if the analyzer is (B) ____________, the battery is (C) ____________ or patient results or analyzer functioning are (D) ____________.
10. A (A) ____________ ____________ is also called a (B) ____________ ____________ after the purified (C) ____________ derivative used in the test.

KNOWLEDGE DRILL 11-2: SCRAMBLED WORDS

1. ampicestie ________________ (microbes in the bloodstream)
2. arcle ________________ (throw this tube away)
3. ayetprint ________________ (test to identify a father)
4. ceatiherput ________________ (beneficial)
5. eclotrane ________________ (capacity to endure without ill effects)
6. gloxticooy ________________ (the study of poisons)
7. guloosotau ________________ (donor and recipient are the same)
8. laedslogycyt ________________ (sugar chemically linked to protein)
9. ralispopdant ________________ (after eating)
10. spitansesi ________________ (prevention of infection by inhibiting microbes)

KNOWLEDGE DRILL 11-3: GLUCOSE TOLERANCE TEST (GTT)

Background: A glucose tolerance test (GTT) is used to diagnose carbohydrate metabolism problems. The major carbohydrate in the blood is glucose, the body's source of energy. The hormone insulin, produced by the pancreas, is primarily responsible for regulating blood glucose levels. The GTT evaluates insulin response to a measured dose of glucose by recording glucose levels on specimens collected at specific time intervals. Results are plotted on a graph, creating what is referred to a GTT curve.

Instructions: The fasting blood glucose for a GTT was collected from a patient at 0500 hours. The blood was tested and the value was normal. The patient was given the glucose drink at 0525 hours and finished drinking it at 0530 hours.

1. Fill in the rest of the GTT collection times in the table below.
2. Using the collection times and the results below, graph the glucose absorption curve.
3. Based on Figure 11-12 and GTT curves in Chapter 11, check which of the following is correct: This graph is

   ________ normal or ________ abnormal.

Timing of GTT	Collection Time	Results
Fasting	0500	75 mg/dL
0.5 hour		250 mg/dL
1.0 hour		200 mg/dL
2.0 hours		175 mg/dL
3.0 hours		150 mg/dL

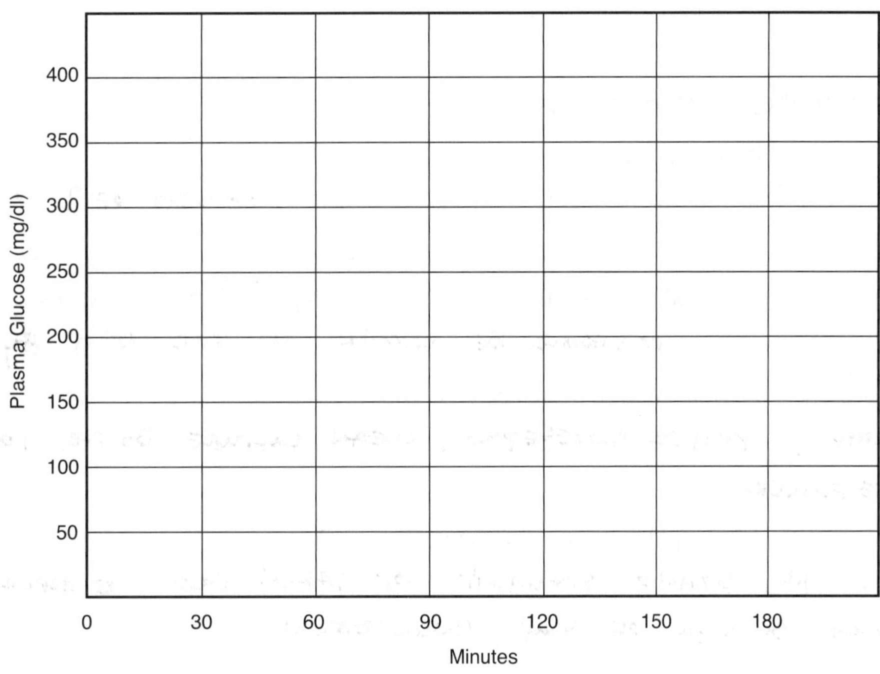

KNOWLEDGE DRILL 11-4: EXAMPLES OF DRUGS NEEDING THERAPEUTIC MONITORING AND THEIR USE

Instructions: Match each DRUG CATEGORY in the middle column below with an EXAMPLE and USE by drawing an arrow between the columns to the appropriate answer. Use a different-colored pen or pencil for each arrow. Answers can be used only once.

Drug Example	Drug Category	Drug Usage
Amikacin	Bronchodilators	Epilepsy
Methotrexate	Protease inhibitors	Bipolar disorder
Tegretol	Anticancer drugs	Asthma
Doxepin	Psychiatric drugs	Psoriasis
Theophylline	Antibiotics	Autoimmune disorders
Digitoxin	Cardiac drugs	Angina
Cyclosporine	Antiepileptics	HIV/AIDS
Atazanavir	Immunosuppressants	Resistant infections

Skills Drills

SKILLS DRILL 11-1: REQUISITION ACTIVITY

Instructions: Answer the following questions concerning the test requisition shown below.

1. How many BC media bottles will be needed to complete this order? 2 SETS OF 2 = 4

2. If the physician wants these blood cultures performed as quickly as possible, how many BCs can be drawn at the same time and from where? IT SHOULD BE DRAWN . ON THE ARM ~~BY~~ MEDIAL 2 CAN BE

3. Describe the special collection technique that must be used before obtaining these samples.
CUBITAL. , PROPER ANTESEPSIS , CLEAN CULTURE BOTTLE TOPS, CLEAN GLOVE FINGER

4. To be more efficient, should the phlebotomist ask the nurse to collect it from the heparin lock that is in the right forearm? Explain. NO, DRAWS SHOULDN'T BE TAKEN FROM THE HEPARIN UNLESS NECESSARY, BECAUSE OF HIGH CONCENTRATION.

Any Hospital USA
1123 West Physician Drive
Any Town USA

Laboratory Test Requisition

PATIENT INFORMATION:

Name: Smith (last) George (first) L (MI)

Identification Number: 09365784 Birth Date: 06/21/75

Referring Physician: Hurstmatson

Date to be Collected: 05/20/12 Time to be Collected: STAT

Special Instructions: need to start antibiotics ASAP

TEST(S) REQUIRED:

____ NH4 – Ammonia	____ Gluc – glucose
____ Bili – Bilirubin, total & direct	____ Hgb – hemoglobin
____ BMP – basic metabolic panel	____ Lact – lactic acid/lactate
____ BUN - Blood urea nitrogen	____ Plt. Ct. – platelet count
____ Lytes – electrolytes	____ PT – prothrombin time
____ CBC – complete blood count	____ PTT – partial thromboplastin time
____ Chol – cholesterol	____ RPR – rapid plasma reagin
____ ESR – erythrocyte sed rate	____ T&S – type and screen
____ EtOH - alcohol	____ PSA – prostate specific antigen
____ D-dimer	Other *blood cultures X 2*

SKILLS DRILL 11-2: WORD BUILDING (See Chapter 4, Medical Terminology)

Divide each of the words below into all of its elements (parts); prefix (P), word root (WR), combining vowel (CV), and suffix (S). Write the word part, its definition, and the meaning of the word on the corresponding lines. If the word does not have a particular element, write NA (not applicable) in its place.

Example: thyrotoxicosis

Elements ______ / *thyr* / *o* / *toxic* / *osis*
P WR CV WR S

Definitions ______ / *thyroid* / ______ / *toxic* / *abnormal condition*

Meaning: abnormal condition of a toxic thyroid gland

1. bacteremia

Elements ______ / ______ / ______ / ______
P WR CV S

Definitions ______ / ______ / ______ / ______

Meaning:

2. hypoglycemic

Elements ______ / ______ / ______ / ______ / ______
P CV WR CV S

Definitions ______ / ______ / ______ / ______ / ______

Meaning:

3. anaerobic

Elements ______ / ______ / ______ / ______ / ______
P CV WR CV S

Definitions ______ / ______ / ______ / ______ / ______

Meaning:

4. antibiotic

Elements ______ / ______ / ______ / ______ / ______
P CV WR CV S

Definitions ______ / ______ / ______ / ______ / ______

Meaning:

5. antimicrobial

Elements ______ / ______ / ______ / ______ / ______
P CV WR CV S

Definitions ______ / ______ / ______ / ______ / ______

Meaning:

6. gastrointestinal

Elements ______ / ______ / ______ / ______ / ______
WR CV WR CV S

Definitions ______ / ______ / ______ / ______ / ______

Meaning:

7. amniocentesis

Elements ______ / ______ / ______ / ______
P WR CV S

Definitions ______ / ______ / ______ / ______

Meaning:

SKILLS DRILL 11-3: BLOOD CULTURE SPECIMEN COLLECTION

Instructions: Match the rationale with the corresponding step in the procedure.

Procedure Step

1. _____ Identify venipuncture site and release tourniquet.
2. _____ Aseptically select and assemble equipment.
3. _____ Perform friction scrub as prescribed.
4. _____ Allow site to air-dry.
5. _____ Cleanse the culture bottle stoppers while the site is drying.
6. _____ Mark the minimum and maximum fill on the culture bottles.
7. _____ Reapply tourniquet and perform venipuncture without touching the site.
8. _____ Inoculate the media bottles as required.
9. _____ Label the specimen containers with required ID, including the site of collection.

Rationale

A. Antisepsis does not occur instantly.
B. Notation of site location is necessary because there may be an isolated infection in that area.
C. Ensuring antiseptic technique and sterility of the site is critical to accurate diagnosis.
D. The CLSI standard states that the tourniquet should not be left on longer than 1 minute.
E. Inoculation of the medium can occur directly into the bottle or after collection when a syringe is used.
F. Blood culture bottles have vacuum, but it is not always measured as in evacuated tubes.
G. Aseptic technique reduces the risk of false positives due to contamination.
H. The tops of the culture bottles must be free of contaminants when they are inoculated.
I. Bacteria exist on the skin surface and can be removed temporarily.

SKILLS DRILL 11-4: RATIONALE FOR BLEEDING TIME PROCEDURE

1. Why are hands sanitized before touching the patient?

____

____

____

2. Why must you determine whether the patient has taken aspirin or other salicylate-containing drugs within the last 2 weeks?

____

____

____

3. Why select the lateral rather than the medial aspect of the arm for the BT?

____

____

____

4. Why should the puncture device blade slot not be touched or rested on any nonsterile surface?

____

____

____

5. Why use a blood pressure cuff and maintain the pressure at 40 mm Hg in this procedure?

____

____

____

6. What is meant by "wicking"? Why is it necessary to "wick" the blood every 30 seconds?

____

____

____

7. Describe how the end point of bleeding-time test is determined.

____

____

____

8. What is the rationale for using a butterfly bandage or Steri Strip following the BT?

____

____

____

SKILLS DRILL 11-5: TB TEST ADMINISTRATION (Text Procedure Box 11-5)

Instructions: Using the TEXTBOOK, fill in the blanks with the missing information.

Step	Rationale
1. Identify the patient, (A) __________ the procedure, and sanitize hands	Correct ID is vital to patient safety and meaningful test results. Proper hand hygiene plays a major role in infection control by protecting the phlebotomist, patient, and others from contamination. Gloves are sometimes put on at this point. Follow facility protocol.
2. Support the patient's arm on a firm surface and select a suitable site on the (B) __________ of the forearm, (C) __________ the antecubital crease.	The arm must be supported to minimize movement during test administration. Areas with scars, bruises, burns, rashes, excessive hair, or superficial veins must be avoided as they can interfere with (D) __________ of the test.
3. Clean the site with an (E) __________ pad and allow it to air dry.	Cleaning with antiseptic and allowing it to air dry permits maximum antiseptic action.

4. Put on gloves at this point if you have not already done so.	Gloves are necessary for safety and infection control.
5. Clean the top of the antigen bottle and draw (F) ____________ of diluted antigen into the syringe.	The top of the bottle must be clean to prevent (G) ______________ of the antigen.
6. Stretch the skin (H) ____________ with the thumb in a manner similar to venipuncture and slip the needle just under the skin at a very (I) ____________ ____________ (approximately 10–15 degrees).	The skin must be taut so that the needle will slip into it easily. The antigen must be injected just (J) __________ ________ ______________ for accurate interpretation of results.
7. Pull (K) ____________ on the syringe plunger slightly to make certain a vein has not been entered.	The antigen must not be injected into a vein.
8. Slowly expel the contents of the syringe to create a distinct, pale elevation commonly called a bleb or (L) ____________.	Appearance of the bleb or wheal is a (M) ____________ that the antigen has been injected properly.
9. Without applying pressure or gauze to the site, withdraw the needle, activate safety feature, and discard the needle.	Applying pressure could force the (N) ____________ out of the site. Gauze might absorb the antigen. Both actions could invalidate test results. Activation of safety features and prompt needle disposal minimizes the chance of an accidental needlestick.
10. Ensure that the arm remains extended until the site has time to close. Do (O) ______ ______ a bandage.	A bandage can absorb the fluid or cause irritation, resulting in misinterpretation of test results.
11. Check the site for a reaction in (P) ____________. This is called "reading" the reaction.	Maximum reaction is achieved in 48–72 hours. A reaction can be underestimated if read after this time.
12. Measure (Q) ____________ (hardness) and interpret the result. Do not measure erythema (redness). *Negative:* induration absent or less than 5 mm in diameter.	A TB reaction is interpreted according to the amount of induration or firm raised area due to (R) ____________. A health status and age of the individual are important considerations when interpreting results.
Doubtful: induration between 5 and 9 mm in diameter. *Positive:* induration (S) ____________ ________ ______________ in diameter.	5 mm of induration can be considered a positive test result in patients who are immunosuppressed due to chronic medical conditions.

SKILLS DRILL 11-6: PREGNANCY TEST PROCEDURE

Instructions: Match the rationale with the corresponding step in the procedure.

Procedure Step

1. _____ Identify the patient according to facility policy.
2. _____ Label the specimen cup with the patient's label.
3. _____ Obtain the patient's urine specimen.
4. _____ Remove the test device from the protective pouch and place it on a flat surface.
5. _____ Using the disposable dropper provided, add 3 drops of sample to the cassette well.
6. _____ Set a timer for the time the kit's manufacturer states a negative test must be read.
7. _____ Read the cassette window's results when the timer goes off.

Rationale

A. To avoid errors, label the specimen even if it is the only one being tested at that time.
B. For correct results, the urine must flow evenly onto the testing surface of the device.
C. The reaction time must be carefully timed and *not read* after 10 minutes.
D. The size of the drops must be exactly as specified and consistent for results to be accurate.
E. Correct ID is vital to patient safety and meaningful test results.
F. If the patient will be collecting a urine specimen at your testing site, explain how to do so.
G. A positive result can be read as soon as lines at both the T and C areas of the test cassette window appear.

Crossword

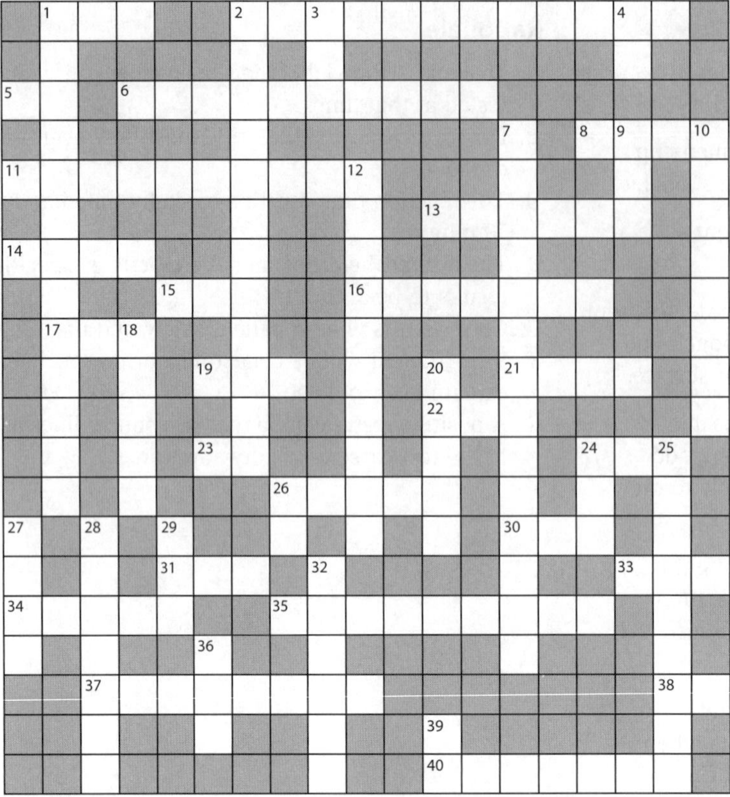

ACROSS

1. Coagulation test used to monitor heparin therapy
2. Increased blood potassium
5. Scientific symbol for mercury
6. Blood types suitable to mix
8. BAC tests for this type of alcohol
11. Blood donated by people who will use it themselves
13. Another name for occult blood testing
14. Institute that defines collection requirements for urine drug screen
15. Company that makes Surgicutt tool
16. Blood bank identification system
17. Type of antimicrobial resin
19. The correct name for a heart attack (abbrev.)
21. Type of Hgb that is measured in blood plasma
22. Quality control built into the instrument (abbrev.)
23. Processes in place to ensure that testing is done properly (abbrev.)
24. Agency that regulates blood products
26. Body fluid excreted by kidneys
30. Approx number of gestational weeks for peak levels of HCG
31. Cardiac protein specific for heart muscle
33. Name of POC chemistry instrument made by IL
34. Handheld POC chemistry analyzer
35. Small, individual POC testing unit for various analytes
37. Type of glucose meter
38. POC test that evaluates platelet function
40. BC media bottle used to grow microbes needing air

DOWN

1. Process of clumping together (i.e., ag–ab reaction)
2. Pertaining to a low glucose level
3. Partial thromboplastin time
4. Identification (abbrev.)
7. Strict protocol for forensic specimens
9. Tight glycemic index
10. Small, portable POCT instruments
12. Microorganisms or their toxins in the blood
18. Volunteer who gives blood for another person's use
20. Body matter/discharge used to test for occult blood
24. Name of charcoal antimicrobial resin bottle (abbrev.)
25. BC media bottle used to grow microbes without air
26. Urinalysis (abbrev.)
27. Law that states qualifications for personnel who do POC testing
28. A 9:1 ratio of blood to this anticoagulant is required
29. Extended test used to diagnose carbohydrate metabolism issues
32. Groups of commonly ordered tests for POCT
36. POCT kidney function test abbrev
39. One of the electrolytes measured by POC instruments

Chapter Review Questions

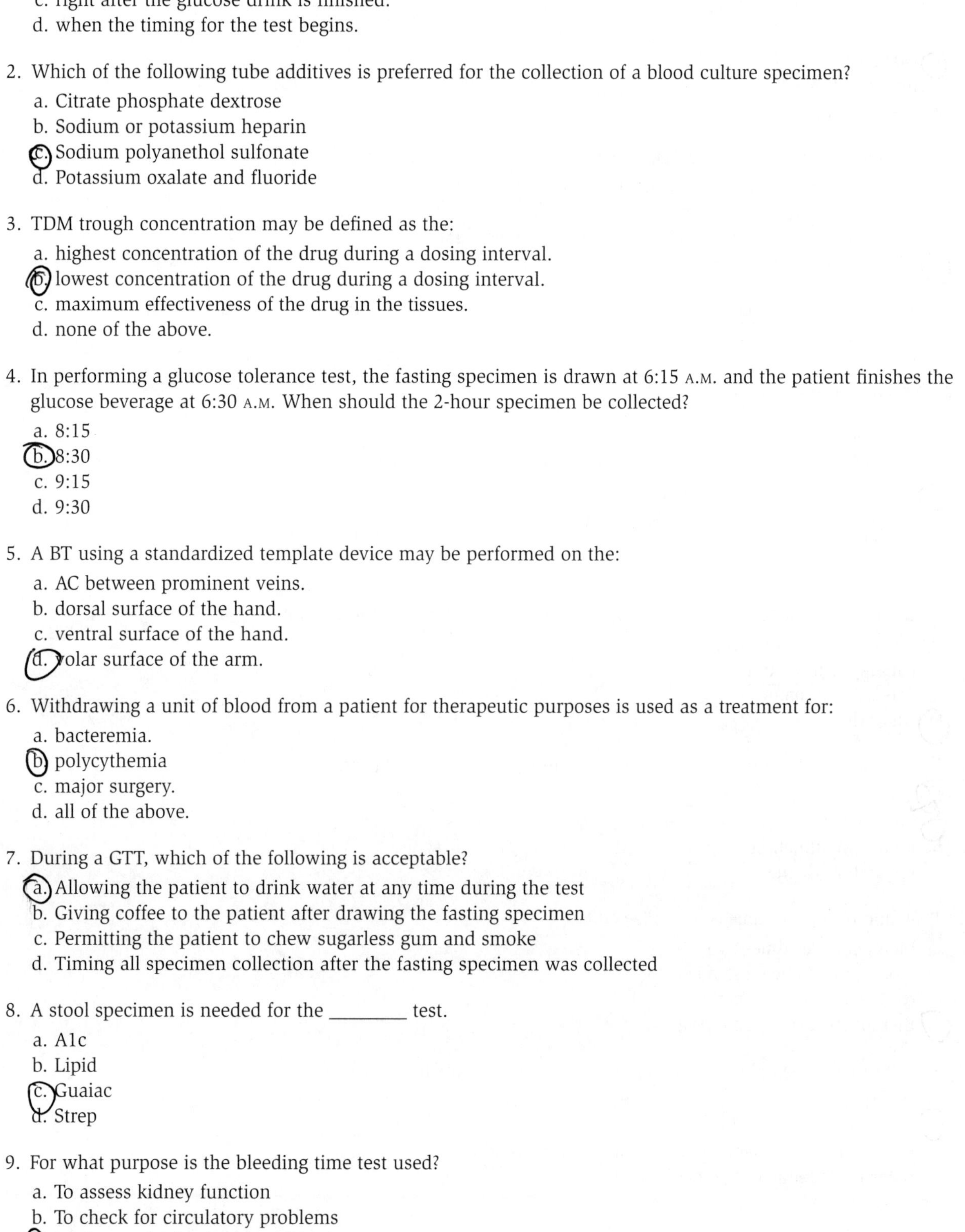

1. The fasting specimen for a GTT is drawn:
   a. as close to 6:00 A.M. as possible.
   b. before the test has actually begun.
   c. right after the glucose drink is finished.
   d. when the timing for the test begins.

2. Which of the following tube additives is preferred for the collection of a blood culture specimen?
   a. Citrate phosphate dextrose
   b. Sodium or potassium heparin
   c. Sodium polyanethol sulfonate
   d. Potassium oxalate and fluoride

3. TDM trough concentration may be defined as the:
   a. highest concentration of the drug during a dosing interval.
   b. lowest concentration of the drug during a dosing interval.
   c. maximum effectiveness of the drug in the tissues.
   d. none of the above.

4. In performing a glucose tolerance test, the fasting specimen is drawn at 6:15 A.M. and the patient finishes the glucose beverage at 6:30 A.M. When should the 2-hour specimen be collected?
   a. 8:15
   b. 8:30
   c. 9:15
   d. 9:30

5. A BT using a standardized template device may be performed on the:
   a. AC between prominent veins.
   b. dorsal surface of the hand.
   c. ventral surface of the hand.
   d. volar surface of the arm.

6. Withdrawing a unit of blood from a patient for therapeutic purposes is used as a treatment for:
   a. bacteremia.
   b. polycythemia
   c. major surgery.
   d. all of the above.

7. During a GTT, which of the following is acceptable?
   a. Allowing the patient to drink water at any time during the test
   b. Giving coffee to the patient after drawing the fasting specimen
   c. Permitting the patient to chew sugarless gum and smoke
   d. Timing all specimen collection after the fasting specimen was collected

8. A stool specimen is needed for the ________ test.
   a. A1c
   b. Lipid
   c. Guaiac
   d. Strep

9. For what purpose is the bleeding time test used?
   a. To assess kidney function
   b. To check for circulatory problems
   c. To detect platelet function disorders
   d. To diagnose diabetes mellitus

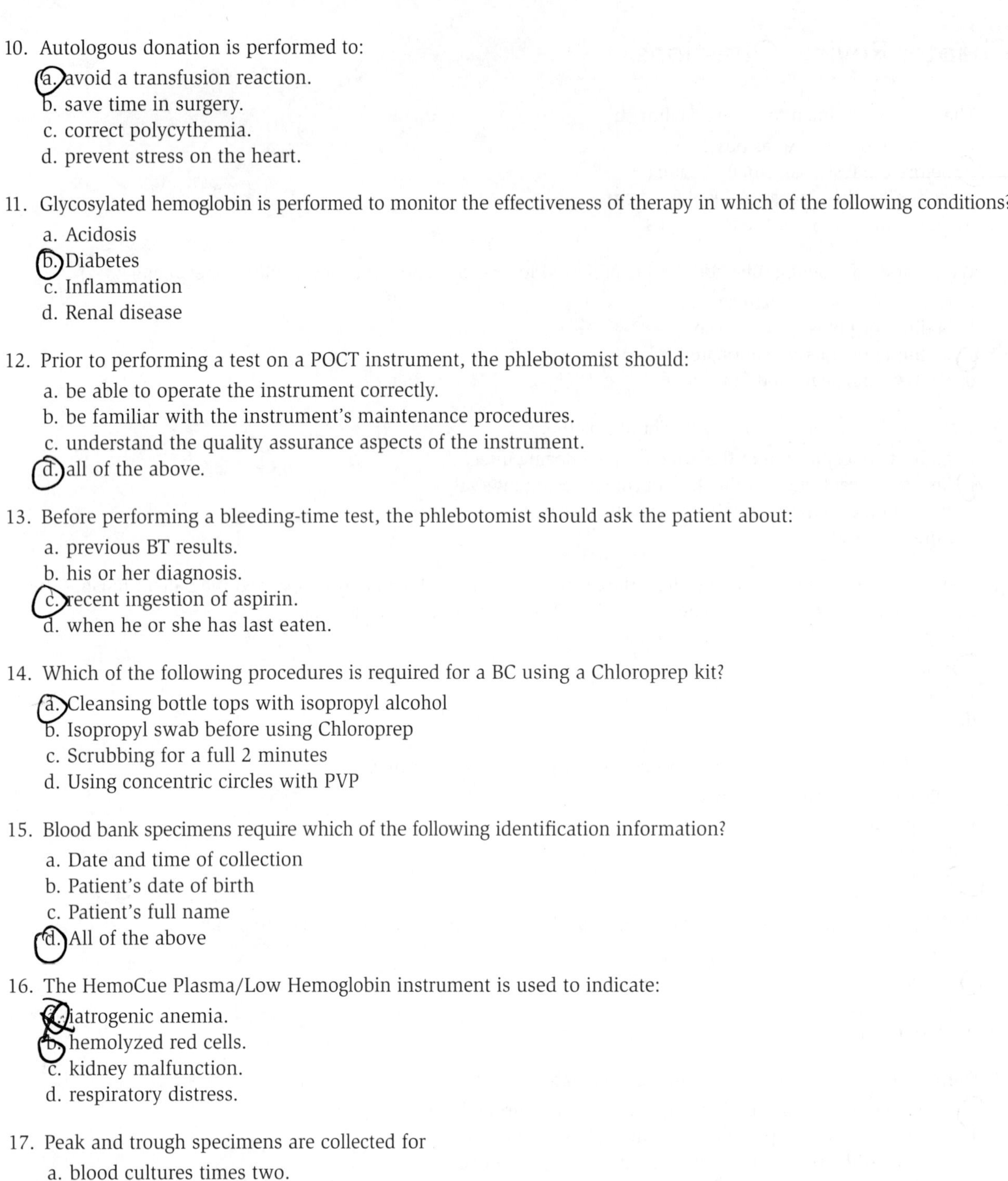

10. Autologous donation is performed to:
   a. avoid a transfusion reaction.
   b. save time in surgery.
   c. correct polycythemia.
   d. prevent stress on the heart.

11. Glycosylated hemoglobin is performed to monitor the effectiveness of therapy in which of the following conditions?
   a. Acidosis
   b. Diabetes
   c. Inflammation
   d. Renal disease

12. Prior to performing a test on a POCT instrument, the phlebotomist should:
   a. be able to operate the instrument correctly.
   b. be familiar with the instrument's maintenance procedures.
   c. understand the quality assurance aspects of the instrument.
   d. all of the above.

13. Before performing a bleeding-time test, the phlebotomist should ask the patient about:
   a. previous BT results.
   b. his or her diagnosis.
   c. recent ingestion of aspirin.
   d. when he or she has last eaten.

14. Which of the following procedures is required for a BC using a Chloroprep kit?
   a. Cleansing bottle tops with isopropyl alcohol
   b. Isopropyl swab before using Chloroprep
   c. Scrubbing for a full 2 minutes
   d. Using concentric circles with PVP

15. Blood bank specimens require which of the following identification information?
   a. Date and time of collection
   b. Patient's date of birth
   c. Patient's full name
   d. All of the above

16. The HemoCue Plasma/Low Hemoglobin instrument is used to indicate:
   a. iatrogenic anemia.
   b. hemolyzed red cells.
   c. kidney malfunction.
   d. respiratory distress.

17. Peak and trough specimens are collected for
   a. blood cultures times two.
   b. blood units to be cross-matched.
   c. cardiac enzyme evaluation.
   d. therapeutic drug monitoring.

18. In collecting blood cultures, one of the most frequent errors made is
   a. failure to inoculate two media bottles
   b. improper cleansing of the site on the arm.
   c. placing an insufficient amount of blood in the bottles.
   d. incorrect labeling of the media bottles.

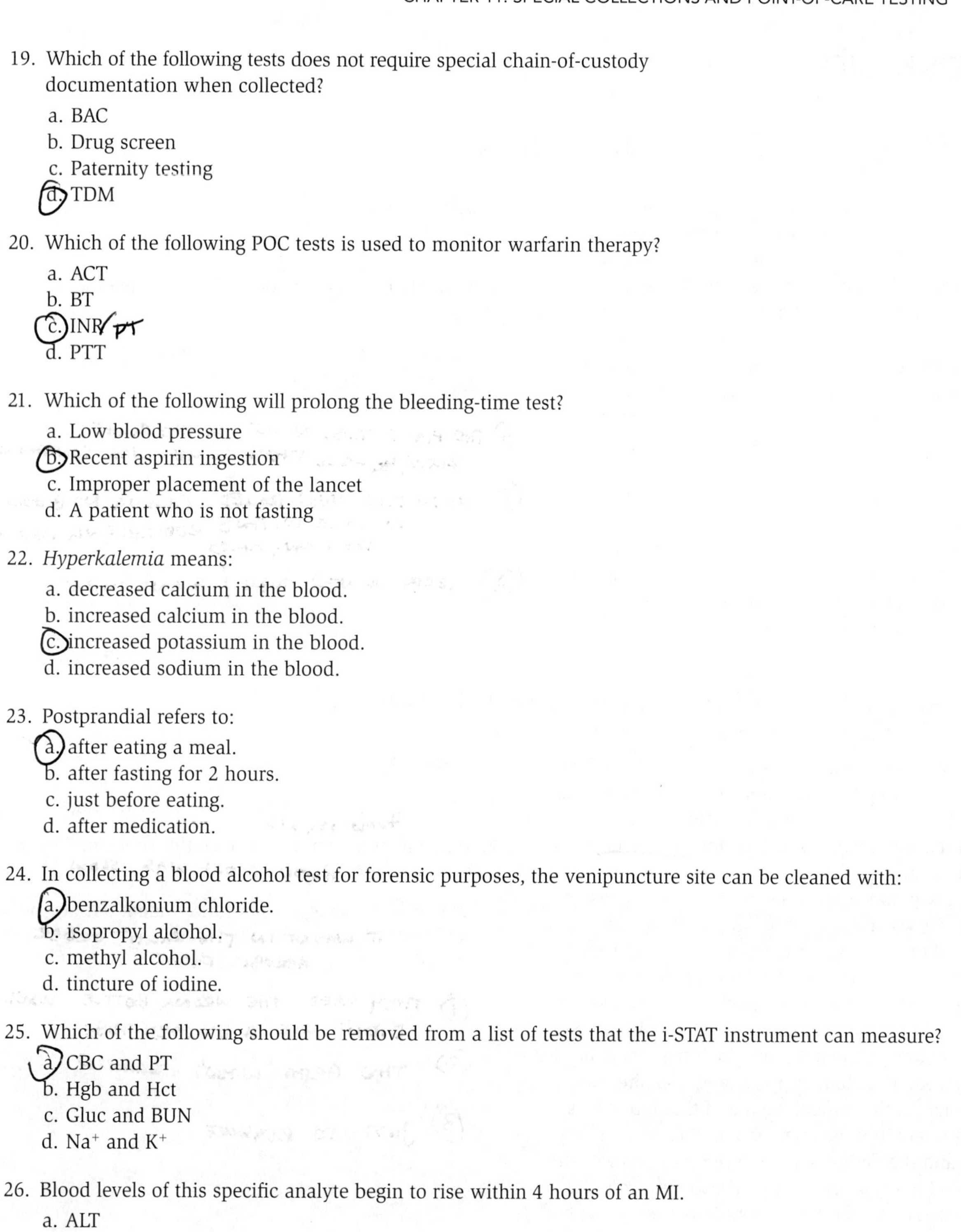

19. Which of the following tests does not require special chain-of-custody documentation when collected?
    a. BAC
    b. Drug screen
    c. Paternity testing
    d. TDM

20. Which of the following POC tests is used to monitor warfarin therapy?
    a. ACT
    b. BT
    c. INR
    d. PTT

21. Which of the following will prolong the bleeding-time test?
    a. Low blood pressure
    b. Recent aspirin ingestion
    c. Improper placement of the lancet
    d. A patient who is not fasting

22. *Hyperkalemia* means:
    a. decreased calcium in the blood.
    b. increased calcium in the blood.
    c. increased potassium in the blood.
    d. increased sodium in the blood.

23. Postprandial refers to:
    a. after eating a meal.
    b. after fasting for 2 hours.
    c. just before eating.
    d. after medication.

24. In collecting a blood alcohol test for forensic purposes, the venipuncture site can be cleaned with:
    a. benzalkonium chloride.
    b. isopropyl alcohol.
    c. methyl alcohol.
    d. tincture of iodine.

25. Which of the following should be removed from a list of tests that the i-STAT instrument can measure?
    a. CBC and PT
    b. Hgb and Hct
    c. Gluc and BUN
    d. Na^+ and K^+

26. Blood levels of this specific analyte begin to rise within 4 hours of an MI.
    a. ALT
    b. TnT
    c. LDL
    d. BNP

CASE STUDIES

Case Study 11-1 Prothrombin Test Collection

During clinical practicum, a phlebotomy student found that the requirements for drawing prothrombin times were not the same as he was taught in class. His clinical coordinator made it very clear that he was to follow facility protocol while he was in his clinical practicum. Therefore, when he was asked to collect a CBC and prothrombin time from a patient, he knew that the order of draw at this facility was citrate first, no discard tube. As he started to draw the specimen from the patient, he immediately ran into trouble when the vein rolled. He was certain that the needle had slipped beside the vein, so he tried to redirect it into the vein. After two unsuccessful redirects, the needle successfully entered the vein. He collected the citrate tube, followed by a lavender-top tube for the CBC. Later that day the coagulation department rejected the specimen and he was sent to re-collect it.

QUESTIONS

1. Why would the lab reject the sample?
2. What had the student done to cause the sample to be rejected?
3. How could the problem have been corrected while the needle was still in the arm?

Case Study 11-2 Blood Cultures and Butterflies

A phlebotomist was acting as preceptor for a phlebotomy student from the local college and was anxious to help her learn all the special tests that had not been practiced in class. When a stat blood culture and lytes on a patient in the ICU were ordered, the preceptor quickly grabbed the student and they headed for the floor. It was clear after looking at the patient that they would have to use a butterfly in a hand vein to collect the test specimens. The preceptor was busy helping the student prepare the site and, while setting out all of the equipment needed, he did not pay close attention to the order in which the media bottles were placed. The student was elated that she was able to access the difficult vein and that blood was flowing freely into the anaerobic bottle. After filling both it and the aerobic bottle to the proper level, she proceeded to draw an SST for electrolytes from the same site. The blood flow was now very slow, with blood entering the tube only a drop at a time. After patiently waiting for the tube to fill, both she and the preceptor were relieved to get finished. Almost immediately after returning to the lab and processing the sample, they were sent back to redraw the electrolytes because the potassium value was too high. Before leaving, the preceptor grabbed more BC equipment because he knew that the BCs would have to be redrawn also.

QUESTIONS

1. What had caused the potassium to be too high?
2. Why might they have expected this problem during the collection?
3. Why did the preceptor have the student redraw the BC also?

Case Study 11-3 Forensic Blood Alcohol Collection

In his first week on the job, a new graduate phlebotomist is called to the ER for a stat blood draw. When he arrives he is told to collect an ETOH. The patient smells heavily of alcohol and the phlebotomist is pretty certain that this is going to be an elevated ETOH with a legal investigation involved. The phlebotomist studied forensic blood alcohol collection in his training program, but this is the first real one he has collected and he is a little unsure of what to do. He remembers that a certain strict protocol is involved and that the site must not be cleaned with alcohol. All he has on his tray other than alcohol preps are a few benzalkonium chloride preps. He decides to use those. Lab protocol says to use an SST for an ETOH level, but he remembers something from his training about drawing a forensic ETOH in a gray top. He decides to draw one of each tube, collecting the SST first. A police officer arrives just as he is finishing and asks for the specimen in the gray-top tube and the accompanying paperwork. The phlebotomist feels relieved and returns to the lab.

QUESTIONS

1. Was the phlebotomist correct in deciding that the ETOH was going to involve an investigation, and what does a forensic collection involve? -GRAY TOP TUBE AND FOLLOW CHAIN OF CUSTODY
2. What is the strict protocol that the phlebotomist remembered from his training and what does it involve? NOT USING ALCHOL
3. Was benzalkonium chloride an acceptable antiseptic to use to collect the specimen?
4. Was it acceptable to draw both an SST and a gray top? ONE FOR HIS PROTCOL AND OTHER FOR FORENSIC

(1) YES

(2) KNOW THE PAITENT IS INTOXICATED AND THAT HIS TEST WOULD BE OFF.

(3) YES, IT WOULDN'T THROW OFF THE TEST

(4) YES.

CHAPTER

12

Computers and Specimen Handling and Processing

OBJECTIVES

Study the information in the textbook that corresponds to each objective to prepare yourself for the activities in this chapter.

1. Define the key terms and abbreviations listed at the beginning of this chapter.
2. Describe components and elements of a computer, identify general computer skills, and define associated computer terminology.
3. Trace the flow of specimens through the laboratory with an information management system.
4. Explain how bar codes are used in healthcare and list information found on a bar code computer label.
5. Describe routine and special specimen handling procedures for laboratory specimens.
6. Identify time constraints and exceptions for delivery and processing of specimens.
7. Identify OSHA-required protective equipment worn when processing specimens.
8. Describe the steps involved in processing the different types of specimens and identify the criteria for specimen rejection.

Matching

Use choices only once unless otherwise indicated.

MATCHING 12-1: KEY TERMS AND DESCRIPTIONS

Match each key term with the *best* description.

Key Terms (1–18)

1. _____ Accession number
2. _____ Aerosol
3. _____ Aliquot
4. _____ Bar code
5. _____ Central processing
6. _____ CPU
7. _____ Centrifuge
8. _____ Cursor
9. _____ Data
10. _____ DOT
11. _____ Enter key
12. _____ FAA
13. _____ Hardware
14. _____ HPC
15. _____ Icon
16. _____ ID code
17. _____ Input
18. _____ Interface

Descriptions (1–18)

A. Central processing unit of a computer
B. Area where specimens are received and prioritized for testing
C. Button on keyboard for data input
D. Computer equipment used to process data
E. Connect for the purpose of interaction
F. Department of Transportation
G. Enter data into a computer
H. Federal Aviation Administration
I. Fine mist of specimen
J. Flashing indicator on the computer screen
K. Handheld PC
L. Image used to represent a program or function on a computer
M. Information collected for analysis or computation
N. Machine that spins blood and other specimens
O. LIS number generated for a specimen when entered into the computer
P. Parallel array of alternately spaced black bars and white spaces
Q. Portion of a specimen used for testing
R. Unique identification for a computer user

Key Terms (19–35)

19. _____ LAN
20. _____ LIS
21. _____ Menu
22. _____ Mnemonic
23. _____ Network
24. _____ Output
25. _____ Password
26. _____ PDA
27. _____ Preanalytical
28. _____ QNS
29. _____ RAM
30. _____ RFID

Descriptions (19–35)

A. Computer screen and keyboard
B. Computers that are linked together for the purpose of sharing resources
C. Identification and tracking system using radio waves
D. Laboratory information system
E. List of options from which a user may choose
F. Local area networks
G. Memory-aiding codes
H. Personal digital assistant
I. Place to preserve information outside of the CPU
J. Prior to testing a sample
K. Programming or coded instruction required to control computer hardware
L. Quantity not sufficient
M. Random-access memory
N. Read-only memory
O. Return of processed information or data to the user or to someone in another location

31. _____ ROM
32. _____ Software
33. _____ Storage
34. _____ Terminal
35. _____ USB drive

P. Secret code that uniquely identifies a person as system user
Q. Universal Serial Bus device used for storing information

MATCHING 12-2: COMPUTER SKILL AND ACTIVITY PERFORMED

Match the computer skill with the activity performed.

Computer Skill

1. _____ Logging on
2. _____ Cursor movement
3. _____ Using icons
4. _____ Entering data
5. _____ Correcting errors
6. _____ Verifying orders
7. _____ Making order inquiries
8. _____ Deleting orders

Activity Performed

The phlebotomist:

A. Enters information where an indicator is flashing. The indicator resets itself when the Enter key is pressed
B. Looks up a test order and cancels it
C. Presses the delete key and types the information again
D. Retrieves information on another test ordered on the same patient
E. Sits down at the computer and enters a password
F. Types in information, presses the Enter key, and checks what has been entered
G. Types in patient information and presses the Enter key
H. Uses the mouse to click on a small image on the screen

MATCHING 12-3: COMPUTER EQUIPMENT AND COMPUTER ELEMENT

Match the computer equipment with the associated computer element.

Computer Equipment

1. _____ Bar code readers
2. _____ CDs
3. _____ Database systems
4. _____ External hard drives
5. _____ Graphics programs
6. _____ Handhelds
7. _____ Keyboards
8. _____ Middleware
9. _____ Modems
10. _____ Monitors
11. _____ Printers
12. _____ Routers
13. _____ Scanners
14. _____ Spreadsheet programs

Computer Element

A. Hardware
B. Software
C. Storage

MATCHING 12-4: SPECIMEN AND TYPE OF PROCESSING

Match the specimen with the type of processing required. Choices may be used more than once.

Specimen

1. A Aldosterone in a red top
2. B Ammonia in a green top
3. A BMP in an SST
4. C CBC in a lavender top
5. A Copper in a nonadditive royal blue top
6. B Electrolytes in a PST
7. B Glucose in an anticoagulant gray top
8. B PT in a light blue top
9. B Zinc in an EDTA royal blue top
10. C Urinalysis specimen

Type of Processing

A. Centrifuge after clotting
B. Centrifuge immediately
C. Do not centrifuge

SERUM - HAVE TO WAIT
PLASMA - RIGHT AWAY

Labeling Exercises

LABELING EXERCISE 12-1: COMPUTER WORK FLOW CHART (Text Fig. 12-3)

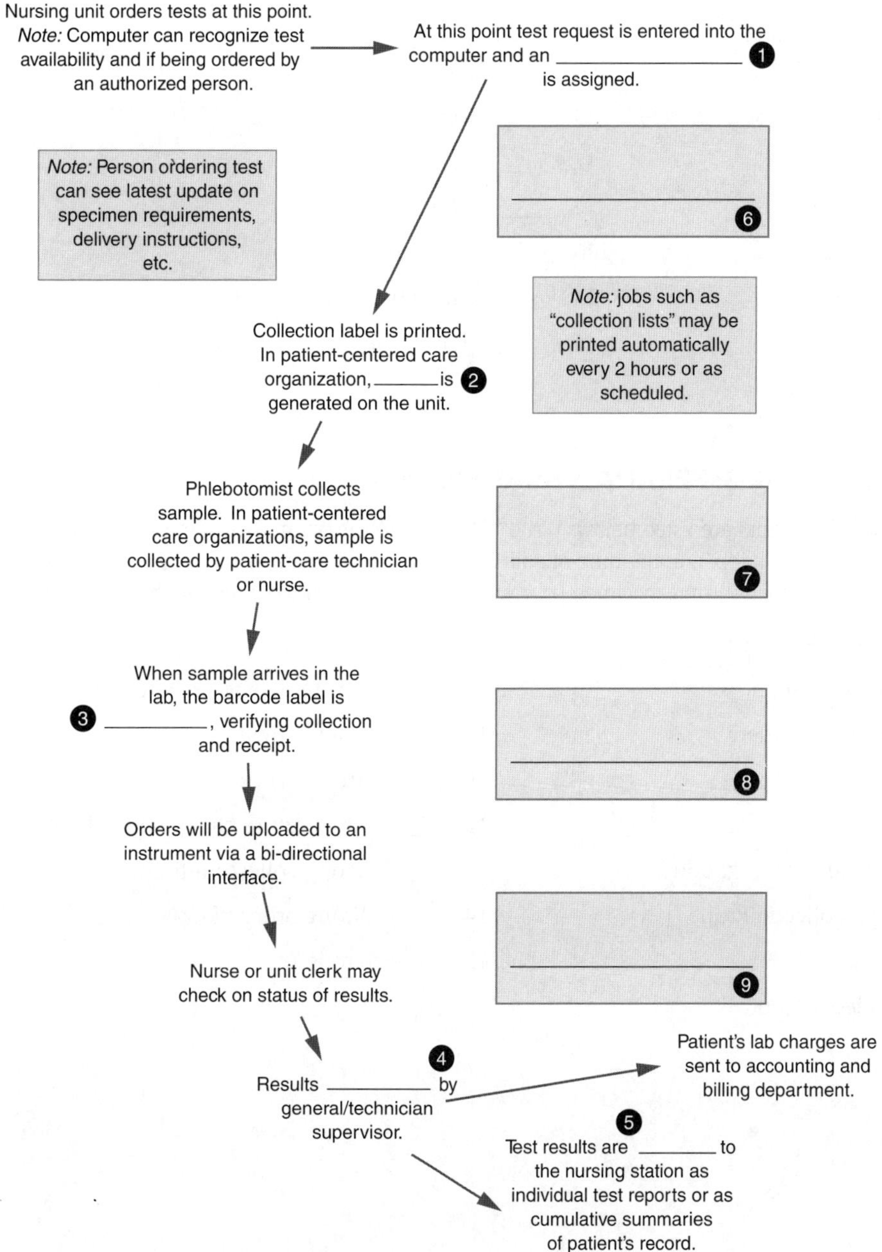

This flow chart describes the test requisition and specimen collection process. Fill in the missing flow chart words numbered 1 through 5 on the corresponding numbered lines. Then write the computer program name of each numbered box in the flow chart on the corresponding numbered line.

1. ________________________
2. ________________________
3. ________________________
4. ________________________
5. ________________________
6. ________________________
7. ________________________
8. ________________________
9. ________________________

LABELING EXERCISE 12-2: SPECIAL HANDLING

Use a blue pen or pencil to place a "C" next to the following specimens that must be chilled in ice slurry. Use a red pen or pencil to place a "W" next to specimens that must be kept warm at 37°C. Use a black pen or pencil to place a "P" next to specimens that must be protected from light.

Tests

1. _____ Acetone
2. _____ Ammonia
3. _____ Bilirubin
4. _____ Carotene
5. _____ Catecholamines
6. _____ Cold agglutinin
7. _____ Cryoglobulin
8. _____ Cryofibrinogen
9. _____ Gastrin
10. _____ Homocysteine
11. _____ Lactic acid
12. _____ Renin
13. _____ Serum folate
14. _____ Urine porphyrins
15. _____ Vitamin B_{12}

LABELING EXERCISE 12-3: PREANALYTICAL ERRORS

Examples of preanalytical errors are listed below. Write "PC" next to the preanalytical errors that happen prior to collection, "TC" next to errors that happen at the time of collection, "ST" next to errors that happen during specimen transport, "SP" next to errors that happen during specimen processing, and "SS" next to errors that happen during specimen storage.

Preanalytical Error Examples

1. _____ Dehydrated patient
2. _____ Duplicate test orders
3. _____ Evaporation
4. _____ Inadequate fast
5. _____ Incomplete centrifugation
6. _____ Incorrect collection tube
7. _____ Medications
8. _____ Mislabeled aliquot
9. _____ Nonsterile site preparation
10. _____ Patient stress
11. _____ Strenuous exercise
12. _____ Temperature change outside of defined limit
13. _____ Wrong collection time
14. _____ Wrong order of draw
15. _____ Wrong test ordered

Knowledge Drills

KNOWLEDGE DRILL 12-1: CAUTION AND KEY POINT RECOGNITION

The following sentences are taken from Caution and Key Point statements found throughout the Chapter 12 text. Using the TEXTBOOK, fill in the blanks with the missing information.

1. (A) ____________ ____________ makes sharing information so easy that (B) ____________ ____________ can be violated.
2. CLSI guideline H18-A3 sets the maximum time limit for (A) ____________ serum and plasma from the (B) ____________ at 2 hours from time of collection unless evidence indicates that a longer contact time will not affect the (C) ____________ of the test result. Less time is recommended for some tests, such as (D) ____________ and potassium.
3. (A) ____________ by erythrocytes and (B) ____________ in blood specimens can falsely lower (C) ____________ values at a rate of up to (D) ____________.
4. (A) ____________ ____________ are factors that alter test results that are introduced into the specimen before testing, including before and during (B)____________, and during (C) ____________, processing, and (D) ____________.
5. It is important to know the following temperatures related to specimen handling:

   Body temperature: (A) ____________

   Room temperature: (B) ____________

   Refrigerated temperature: (C) ____________

   Frozen temperature: (D) ____________ (some specimens require −70°C or lower)
6. (A) ____________ regulations require those who process specimens to wear (B) ____________ ____________ ____________ (________), which includes gloves, fully closed, (C) ____________ resistant lab coats or aprons, and protective face gear, such as mask and goggles with (D) ____________, or chin-length face shields.
7. Stoppers should also be left on tubes during (A) ____________ to prevent (B) ____________, evaporation, (C) ____________ (fine spray) formation, and (D) ____________ changes.
8. Because a centrifuge generates (A) ____________ during operation, specimens requiring (B) ____________ should be processed in a temperature-controlled (C) ____________ centrifuge.
9. Some specimens are negatively affected by (A) ____________. For example, potassium levels artificially increase if the specimen is (B) ____________. When a potassium test is ordered with other analytes that require (C) ____________, it should be collected in a separate tube.
10. Never put (A) ____________ and (B) ____________, or (C) ____________ from specimens with different (D) ____________ in the same aliquot tube.
11. There are different (A) ____________ formulations, and some of them cannot be used for certain tests. For example, (B) ____________ cannot be used for (C) ____________ levels, ammonium (D) ____________ cannot be used for ammonia levels, and sodium (E) ____________ cannot be used for sodium levels.
12. (A) ____________ the serum or plasma into (B) ____________ ____________ is not recommended because it increases the possibility of (C) ____________ formation or (D) ____________.

KNOWLEDGE DRILL 12-2: SCRAMBLED WORDS

Unscramble the following words using the hints given in parenthesis. Write the correct spelling of the scrambled word on the line next to it.

1. cremtoup: ______________________ (healthcare tool)
2. dolttec: ______________________ (SSTs before they can be centrifuged)
3. fewtoras: ______________________ (coded instructions to control hardware)
4. legtangutia: ______________________ (some specimens do this at room temperature)
5. paveroontia: ______________________ (concentrates analytes)
6. pratmeertue: ______________________ (can affect specimen integrity)
7. scisyllogy: ______________________ (metabolic process)
8. sloymeshi: ______________________ (reason for specimen rejection)
9. teeptip: ______________________ (used to create an aliquot)
10. inmalter: ______________________ (a monitor and a keyboard)

KNOWLEDGE DRILL 12-3: SPECIMEN REJECTION CRITERIA

The following are examples of specimen rejection criteria (text Box 12-2). Fill in the blanks with the missing information.

1. Inadequate, (A) __________, or missing specimen (B) __________ (e.g., a urine specimen that is not labeled)
2. (A) __________ tubes containing an inadequate (B) __________ of blood (e.g., a partially filled coagulation tube)
3. Hemolysis (e.g., a [A] __________ specimen intended for [B] __________ determination)
4. Wrong (A) __________ (e.g., a CBC specimen collected in a [B] __________ top tube)
5. (A) __________ tube (e.g., a CBC specimen collected in a tube that [B] __________ the week before)
6. Improper (A) __________ (e.g., a lavender top drawn for a CBC that has [B] __________ in it due to improper [C] __________)
7. (A) __________ specimen (e.g., a urine for culture and sensitivity in an [B] __________ container)
8. (A) __________ specimen, referred to as (B) " __________ not sufficient" (QNS) for the test ordered (e.g., a specimen for an erythrocyte sedimentation rate submitted in a microtainer)
9. Wrong collection (A) __________ (e.g., a specimen for [B] __________ collected before the drug has been given)
10. Exposure to (A) __________ (e.g., [B] __________ results can be 50% lower after 1 hour of exposure to light)
11. Delay in (A) __________ (e.g., a specimen for a [B] __________ in an EDTA tube is only stable for 4 hours at room temperature, and 12 hours if refrigerated, and specimens older than 4 hours will give incorrect PTT results)
12. Delay or error in (A) __________. Serum tubes that have not been spun within 2 hours or (B) __________ of serum tubes before (C) __________ will increase some analytes, such as potassium, creatinine, phosphorus, and LDH, and decrease analytes such as glucose, ionized calcium, and CO_2.

Skills Drills

SKILLS DRILL 12-1: REQUISITION ACTIVITY

Any Hospital USA
1123 West Physician Drive
AnyTown USA

Laboratory Test Requisition

PATIENT INFORMATION:

Name: Doe (last) Jane (first) A (MI)

Identification Number: 713562941 Birth Date: 04/23/40

Referring Physician: Bright, Samuel

Date to be Collected: 08/11/2011 Time to be Collected: 0600

Special Instructions: ______

TEST(S) ORDERED:

Chemistry		**Coagulation**	
	NH4 – Ammonia		D-dimer
√	Bili – Bilirubin, total & direct	√	PT – prothrombin time
	BMP – basic metabolic panel		PTT – partial thromboplastin time
	BUN - Blood urea nitrogen	**Hematology**	
	Chol – cholesterol		CBC – (complete blood count)
	EtOH - alcohol		ESR – (erythrocyte sed rate)
	Gluc – glucose		Hgb – (hemoglobin)
	Lytes – electrolytes		H & H (hemoglobin & Hematocrit)
	Lact – lactic acid/lactate		RBC (Red blood cell count)
	PSA – prostatic specific antigen		WBC (White blood cell count)
Other	√ Cold agglutinin		

A phlebotomist collected specimens for this requisition and delivered them to the specimen processing. One specimen was wrapped in foil; one was in a 37°C heat block, and one was a normal draw light-blue–top tube with no special handling that was about two-thirds full with a note attached stating that it was a difficult draw. The specimens were correctly labeled. Assuming the specimens were handled properly:

1. Which specimen was wrapped in foil? Why? What process does the foil prevent? ______

2. Which specimen was in the heat block? Why? ______

3. Which specimen was in the light blue top? Why? ______

4. Should the light blue top be accepted for testing? Why or why not? ______

SKILLS DRILL 12-2: WORD BUILDING

Divide each of the words below into all of its elements (parts); prefix (P), word root (WR), combining vowel (CV), and suffix (S). Write the word part, its definition, and the meaning of the word on the corresponding lines. If the word does not have a particular element, write NA (not applicable) in its place.

Example: phlebotomy

Elements ______________ / *phleb* / *o* / *tomy*
P WR CV S

Definitions ______________ / *vein* / ____ / *cutting/incision*

Meaning: cutting or incision of a vein

1. glycolysis

Elements ______________ / ______________ / ____ / ______________
P WR CV S

Definitions ______________ / ______________ / ____ / ______________

Meaning:

2. cryofibrinogen

Elements ____________ / ________ / ________ / ____________ / ____________
WR CV WR CV S

Definitions ____________ / ________ / ________ / ____________ / ____________

Meaning:

3. diagnosis

Elements ______________ / ______________ / ____ / ______________
P WR CV S

Definitions ______________ / ______________ / ____ / ______________

Meaning:

4. terminology

Elements ______________ / ______________ / ____ / ______________
P WR CV S

Definitions ______________ / ______________ / ____ / ______________

Meaning:

5. mnemonic

Elements ______________ / ______________ / ____ / ______________
P WR CV S

Definitions ______________ / ______________ / ____ / ______________

Meaning:

6. preanalytical

Elements ______________ / ______________ / ____ / ______________
P WR CV S

Definitions ______________ / ______________ / ____ / ______________

Meaning:

Crossword

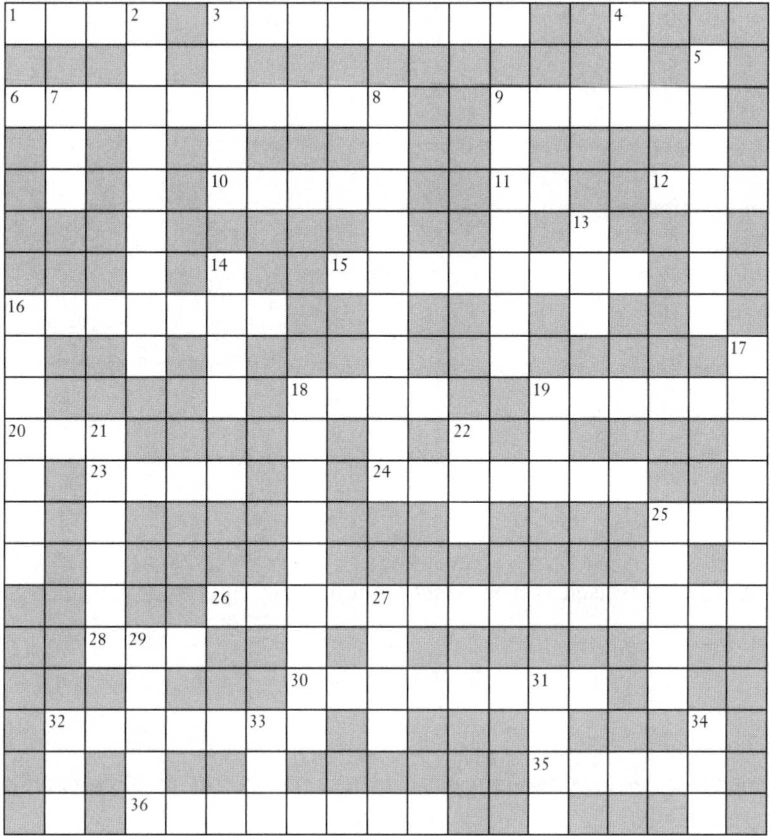

ACROSS

1. Information that has been collected for analysis and computation
3. Another name for the sample being tested
6. Of or relating to electrons
9. Fluid portion of living blood
10. Electronic equipment used to connect computers by telephone line
11. Patient identification (abbrev.)
12. Time from collection to result (abbrev.)
15. Process of using a mechanical device made to duplicate human function
16. Blood spray when tube stopper is removed
18. List of options from which the user may choose
19. To be formed into ice
20. Abbreviation for less than the amount needed
23. Computer terminal is called ____________ ware
24. Place for keeping data (e.g., USB drive)
25. Cardiopulmonary resuscitation
26. Process of spinning blood tube at high rpms
28. Test for diffuse coagulation throughout the body (abbrev.)
30. Device that computes
32. Method of doing something in stepwise procedure
35. Collection vials
36. Coded instructions to control hardware

DOWN

2. Record sample information in the order received
3. Fluid in a clotted tube
4. Computer software system used in the laboratory (abbrev.)
5. Crucial consideration when loading a centrifuge
7. Local interconnected computer network
8. Three basic operations of a computer system
9. Computer peripheral used to create hard copies
13. Substance used to make slurry for chilling specimens
14. Abbreviation used for purposes of tracking specimen
16. Portion of specimen used for testing
17. Anticoagulant in green top tube
18. Memory-aiding abbreviations
19. Agency that regulates packaging on airlines
21. Protective covering or structure
22. Read-only memory (abbrev.)
25. Make specimen cold to slow down metabolic processes
27. Way to measure centrifuge speed (abbrev.)
29. Images used to request appropriate computer functions
31. Anticoagulant in lavender tubes
32. Plasma tubes with separator gel (abbrev.)
33. Serum tubes with separator gel (abbrev.)
34. Test measuring rate of RBC sedimentation (abbrev.)

Chapter Review Questions

1. The abbreviation for computer memory that can be lost if not saved is:
   a. RAM.
   b. REM.
   c. RIM.
   d. ROM.

2. Normal operation of a computer is controlled by:
   a. applications software.
   b. hardware.
   c. storage memory.
   d. systems software.

3. Input devices include:
   a. cursors.
   b. glidepads.
   c. icons.
   d. PDAs.

4. This device automatically resets itself at the correct point for data input after the Enter key is pressed.
   a. cpu
   b. cursor
   c. icon
   d. interface

5. What is the next thing to happen after a specimen is delivered to a lab that has a computerized information system?
   a. A computer interface signals the appropriate instrument.
   b. An accession number is generated and assigned.
   c. The bar code is scanned to verify the collection.
   d. The patient's lab charges are sent to the billing office.

6. Information in the form of alternately spaced black bars and white spaces is called a/an:
   a. accession number.
   b. bar code.
   c. ID code.
   d. mnemonic.

7. The abbreviation of the organization that was established to ensure that POC analyzers are able to talk to any LIS is:
   a. CIC.
   b. CLIA.
   c. DOT.
   d. HIPAA.

8. Results of a bilirubin test specimen exposed to light for an hour can be decreased up to:
   a. 10%.
   b. 25%.
   c. 50%.
   d. 65%.

9. Glycolysis can falsely lower glucose values at a rate of up to:
   a. 10 mg/L per hour.
   b. 100 mg/L per hour.
   c. 200 mg/L per hour.
   d. 500 mg/L per hour.

10. Inadequate mixing of an anticoagulant tube can lead to:
    a. aerosol formation.
    b. glycolysis.
    c. hemolysis.
    d. microclot formation.

11. Normal body temperature is:
    a. 20°F.
    b. 37°C.
    c. 37°F.
    d. 98.6°C.

12. The specimen for this test should not be chilled.
    a. Ammonia
    b. Homocysteine
    c. Lactic acid
    d. Potassium

13. To "balance" a centrifuge means to:
    a. put tubes of equal size and amount of specimen opposite each other.
    b. fill it completely with tubes that are all of the same specimen type.
    c. place it on a sturdy countertop with a level and motionless surface.
    d. all of the above.

14. Which of the following actions by a specimen processor violates OSHA regulations?
    a. Loading specimens into the centrifuge without wearing gloves
    b. Pouring specimens into aliquot tubes instead of using pipettes
    c. Wearing an unfastened lab coat while creating specimen aliquots
    d. All of the above

15. Latent fibrin formation in serum can result from:
    a. a centrifuge speed that is set too high.
    b. a long delay before centrifugation.
    c. clotting incomplete when centrifuged.
    d. gross hemolysis of the specimen.

16. Which specimen should not be centrifuged?
    a. CBC
    b. Glucose
    c. Protime
    d. Vitamin B_{12}

17. Which of the following would most likely be rejected for testing?
    a. Bilirubin specimen in a half-fille microtube
    b. CBC specimen in a slightly underfilled tube
    c. Hemolyzed specimen for potassium testing
    d. UA specimen in a container that is not sterile

18. Which specimen may take longer than normal to clot?
    a. Chilled specimen that is from an outpatient clinic
    b. Specimen from a patient with a high WBC count
    c. Specimen from a patient on anticoagulant therapy
    d. All of the above

CASE STUDIES

Case Study 12-1 Specimen Handling and Collection Verification

Chad is the lone phlebotomist on the night shift at a hospital. At 0300 he collects a timed glucose using a PST per lab policy. On return to the lab he attempts to verify collection of the specimen. The LIS is down for scheduled updates but will be back on-line soon. He sets the tube in a rack of extra tubes collected during ER draws. He intends to verify collection in a few minutes but starts sorting morning draw requisitions and forgets about it. After that he goes on break and loses track of time reading a newspaper until he is paged by an ER nurse to collect a STAT CBC. He tries but is unable to collect it, so an ER tech collects it while starting an IV. It is past time for Chad's shift to be over, so he quickly grabs the tube, labeling it on the way back to the lab. The 0700 shift is already there. One of them has just returned from trying to collect a glucose specimen because the patient's nurse had called for results and there was no record of the draw. The patient insisted he had already been drawn, and refused to be drawn again. Chad remembers the glucose specimen in the rack. He quickly verifies collection of it and the STAT and personally delivers them to the proper lab departments. The chemistry tech refuses to accept the glucose specimen. When the STAT CBC is tested, microclots are detected, and it has to be recollected.

QUESTIONS

1. Why do you think the glucose specimen was rejected for testing?
2. What could Chad have done differently so the specimen would not have been forgotten?
3. What do you think caused the microclots in the CBC?
4. How should Chad have handled the CBC?

Case Study 12-2 Specimen Rejection and Centrifuge Operation

Melinda, a recent phlebotomy graduate, works with an experienced phlebotomist in a clinic. Her job involves drawing specimens, centrifuging them if required, and sending them by courier to an off-site lab. Today her coworker is ill, and Melinda is by herself. Quite a few patients arrived shortly after the clinic opened at 0800, but most were easy draws and by 0915 only three are left. The first one, an elderly man, needs a PT and BMP. She draws a light blue top and SST. The next one needs a liver profile. He is a difficult draw and her first attempt is unsuccessful. On the second try blood flows slowly, but she is able to collect a few milliliters in an SST before it stops. The last patient needs a homocysteine level. She easily draws a lavender top. The waiting room is empty. She looks at the clock. It is 0940. The courier arrives in 20 minutes and she has not centrifuged any of the specimens. She quickly loads the centrifuge and turns it on. It makes a terrible noise so she turns it off. She moves a few tubes around and starts it again. This time it sounds OK and finishes spinning just as the courier arrives. She quickly grabs the tubes. As she puts them in a transport bag, she notices the serum in one SST looks gelled. She wonders why, but puts it in the bag anyway. The courier takes the bag and leaves. The elderly man's BMP specimen, the difficult draw specimen, and the homocysteine specimen are all rejected by the lab and must be recollected.

QUESTIONS

1. Why do you think the centrifuge made the noise? Why did moving tubes fix the problem?
2. What do you think the gel-like substance in the elderly man's BMP specimen was? What may have caused it, and would that be why it was rejected for testing?
3. What do you think was most likely wrong with the difficult draw specimen?
4. Why do you think the homocysteine specimen was rejected?

CHAPTER

13

Nonblood Specimens and Tests

OBJECTIVES

Study the information in your textbook that corresponds to each objective to prepare yourself for the activities in this chapter.

1. Define the key terms and abbreviations listed at the beginning of the chapter.
2. Describe nonblood specimen labeling and handling.
3. Name and describe the various urine tests, specimen types, and collection and handling methods.
4. Identify and describe the types of nonblood specimens other than urine and explain why these specimens are tested.
5. Describe collection and handling procedures indicated for nonblood specimens other than urine.
6. Identify tests performed on various nonblood specimens other than urine.

Matching

Use choices only once unless otherwise indicated.

MATCHING 13-1: KEY TERMS AND DESCRIPTIONS

Match each key term with the *best* description.

Key Terms (1–14)

1. _____ AFP
2. _____ Amniotic fluid
3. _____ Buccal swab
4. _____ C&S
5. _____ *C. difficile*
6. _____ Catheterized
7. _____ Clean-catch
8. _____ CSF
9. _____ expectorate
10. _____ FOBT
11. _____ Gastric analysis
12. _____ *H. pylori*
13. _____ Iontophoresis
14. _____ Midstream

Descriptions (1–14)

A. Antigen in amniotic fluid measured to assess fetal development
B. Bacteria that can cause chronic gastritis and lead to peptic ulcer disease
C. Contains material collected from the inside of the cheek
D. Cough up and spit out mucus or phlegm
E. Detects hidden blood in feces
F. Fluid from the cavity surrounding the brain spinal cord
G. Frequent causative agent of hospital-acquired diarrhea
H. Involves growing and determining the antibiotic susceptibility of a microbe
I. Liquid from the sac that surrounds and cushions a fetus
J. Method of obtaining an uncontaminated urine sample
K. Method used to stimulate sweat production
L. Term for a urine specimen obtained during the middle of urination
M. Test that evaluates stomach acid production
N. Type of urine specimen collected from tubing inserted into the bladder

Key Terms (15–28)

15. _____ NP
16. _____ O&P
17. _____ occult blood
18. _____ pericardial fluid
19. _____ peritoneal fluid
20. _____ pleural fluid
21. _____ serous fluid
22. _____ sputum
23. _____ suprapubic
24. _____ sweat chloride
25. _____ synovial fluid
26. _____ 24-hour urine
27. _____ UA
28. _____ UTI

Descriptions (15–28)

A. Blood hidden from the naked eye
B. Fecal test for parasites and their eggs
C. Fluid from the abdominal cavity
D. Fluid that surrounds the lungs
E. Fluid from the sac surrounding the heart
F. Urinary tract infection
G. Joint fluid
H. Mucus coughed up from the trachea, bronchi, or lungs
I. Pale-yellow serumlike fluid
J. Referring to the nasal cavity and pharynx
K. Routine urine test
L. Test used in the diagnosis of cystic fibrosis
M. Timed urine specimen collected over a 24-hour period
N. Type of urine specimen aspirated through the bladder wall

MATCHING 13-2: NONBLOOD TESTS AND TYPES OF SPECIMENS

Match the test to the type of specimen required.

Nonblood Test

1. _____ AFP
2. _____ Diphtheria culture
3. _____ Guaiac
4. _____ HCG
5. _____ Male fertility studies
6. _____ TB culture

Type of Specimen

A. Amniotic fluid
B. Feces
C. NP swab
D. Semen
E. Sputum
F. Urine

MATCHING 13-3: NONBLOOD TESTS AND TEST EQUIPMENT, PROCEDURES, OR SPECIMEN REQUIREMENTS

Match each of the following nonblood tests to the equipment, procedure, or specimen requirement listed.

Nonblood Test

1. _____ CSF analysis
2. _____ C-urea breath test
3. _____ Gastric analysis
4. _____ NP culture
5. _____ Occult blood
6. _____ Pregnancy test
7. _____ Sweat chloride
8. _____ Urine C&S
9. _____ Urine chemical analysis

Test Equipment, Procedure, or Specimen Requirements

A. Concentrated urine specimen
B. Cotton- or Dacron-tipped flexible wire swab
C. Histamine or pentagastrin as a stimulant
D. Machine with electrodes to stimulate the skin
E. Special Mylar balloons
F. Reagent strip
G. Special card for specimen collection
H. Sterile collection container
I. Three sterile tubes

Labeling Exercises

LABELING EXERCISE 13-1: SPECIMEN CONTAINERS

Label the photo of each specimen container shown below with the name of a test that is collected in it. Choose from the following list of tests.

Tests

AFB culture
Creatinine clearance
O&P
Strep culture
Urine C&S

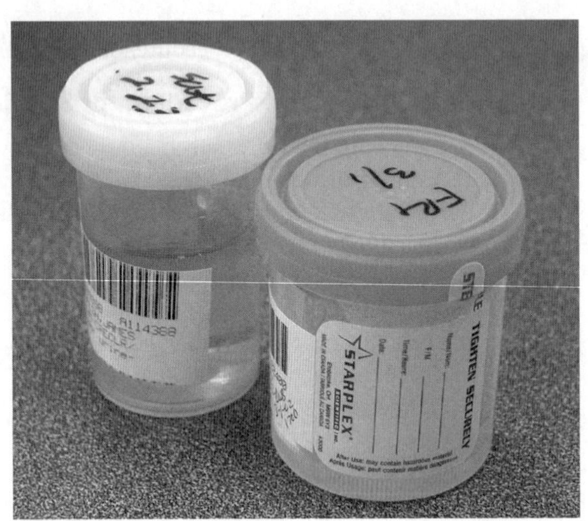

1. ______________________________

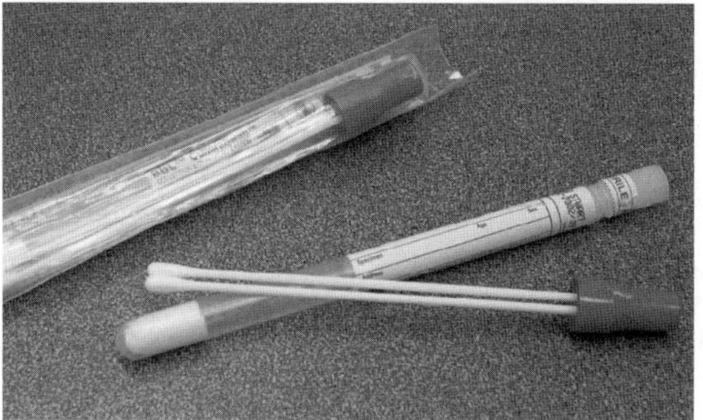

2. ________________________________

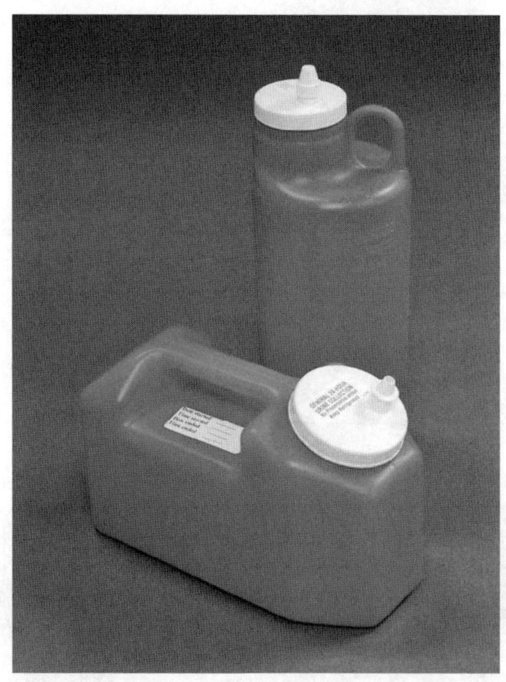

3. ________________________________

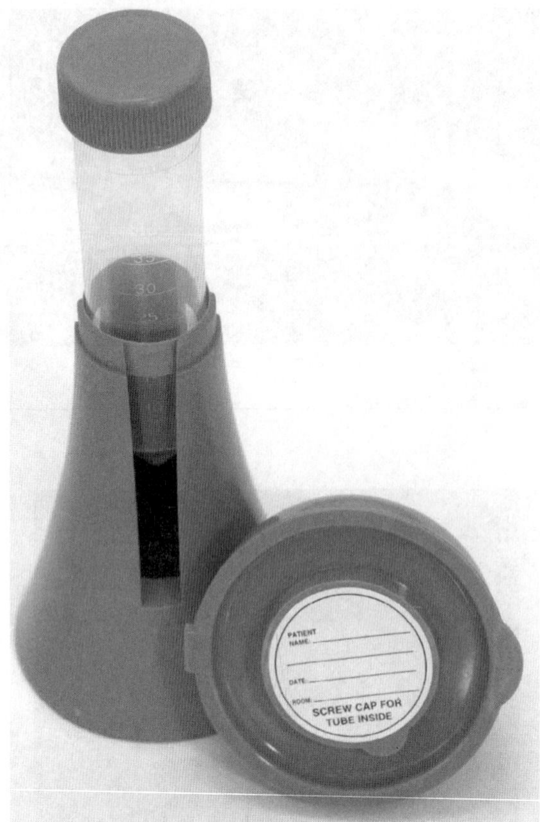
PATIENT NAME
DATE
ROOM
SCREW CAP FOR TUBE INSIDE

4. ______________________________

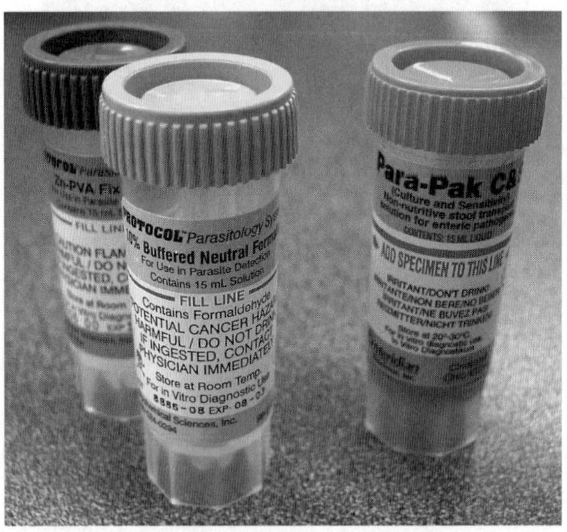
FILL LINE
For Use in Parasite Detection
Contains 15 mL Solution
FILL LINE
Contains Formaldehyde
Store at Room Temp.
(Culture and Sensitivity)
CONTENTS: 15 ML LIQUID
IRRITANT/DON'T DRINK
Store at 20°-30°C

5. ______________________________

LABELING EXERCISE 13-2: BODY FLUIDS

Identify the type of fluid that comes from each numbered area of the body sections illustrated below. Write the name of the fluid on the corresponding line.

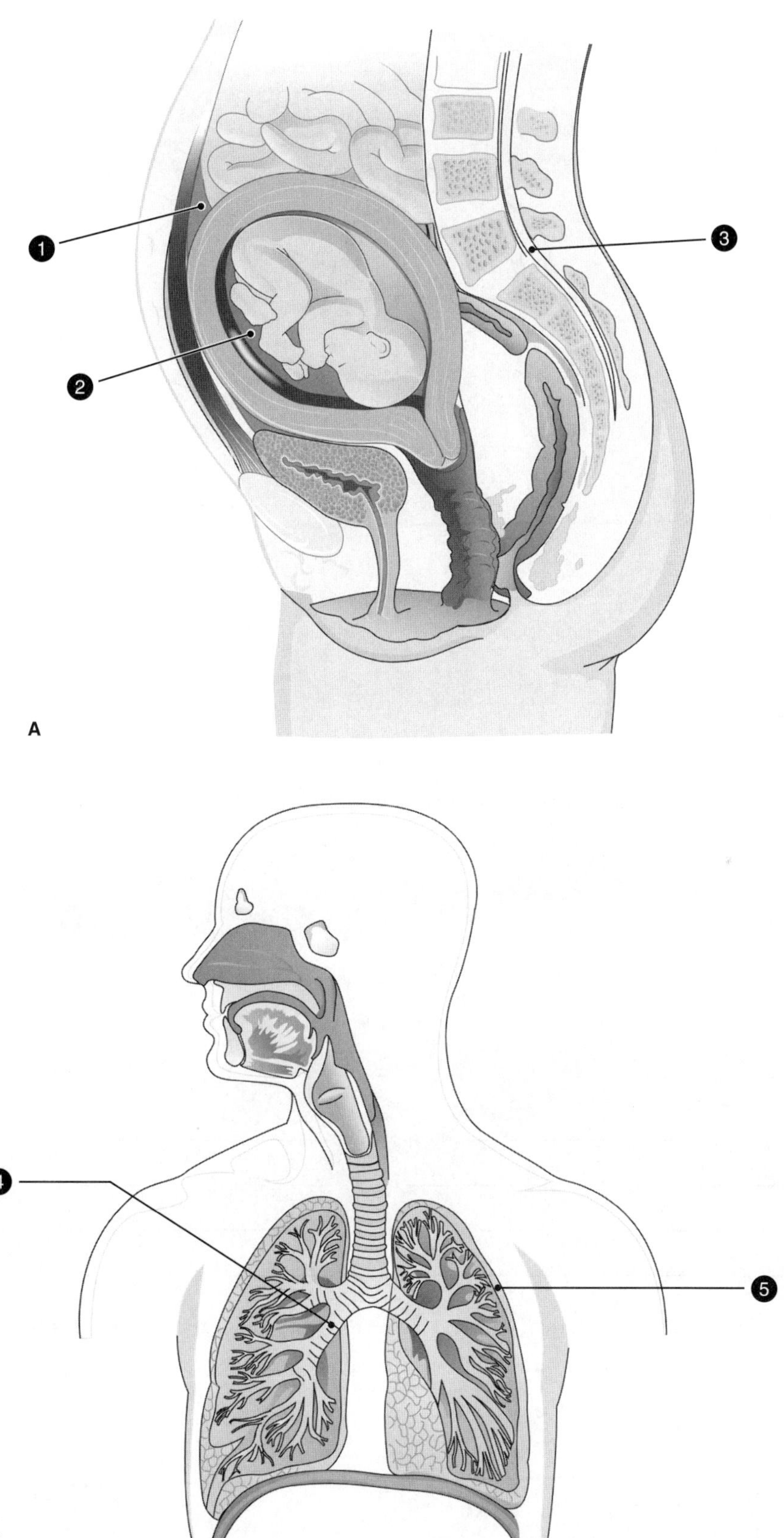

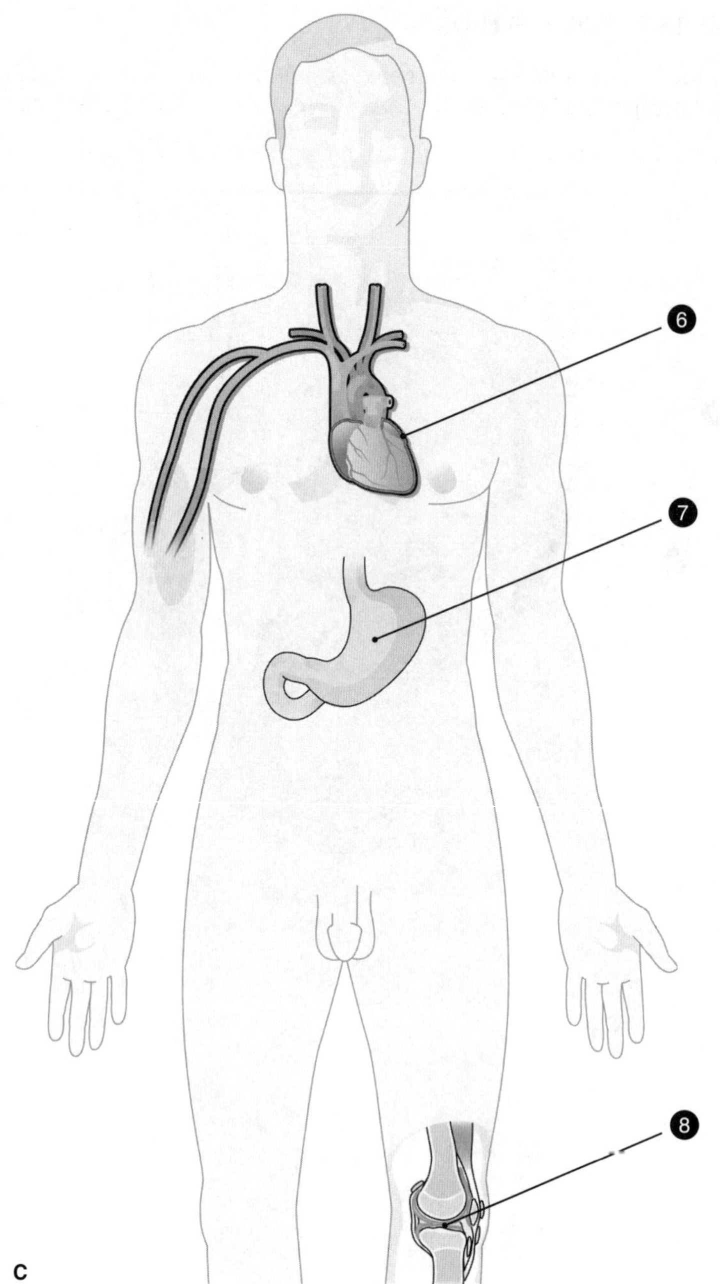

1. ______________________
2. ______________________
3. ______________________
4. ______________________
5. ______________________
6. ______________________
7. ______________________
8. ______________________

Knowledge Drills

KNOWLEDGE DRILL 13-1: CAUTION AND KEY POINT RECOGNITION

The following sentences are taken from Caution and Key Point statements found throughout the Chapter 13 text. Using the TEXTBOOK, fill in the blanks with the missing information.

1. Phlebotomists are often asked to (A) ___________ specimens to the (B) ___________ that have been (C) ___________ by other healthcare personnel. It is important for the phlebotomist to verify proper (D) ___________ before (E) ___________ a specimen for transport.
2. If (A) ___________ specimens are not (B) ___________ promptly, urine (C) ___________ can change. For example, (D) ___________ elements (E) ___________, bilirubin breaks down to (F) ___________, and bacteria multiply, leading to erroneous test results.
3. Specimens for (A) ___________ and other (B) ___________ studies should be transported to the lab and processed (C) ___________. If a delay in transportation or processing is unavoidable the specimen should be (D) ___________.
4. A (A) ___________ specimen should not be collected in a (B) ___________ unless it is one specifically designed for specimen collection. Regular (C) ___________ often contain (D) ___________ (substances that [E] ___________ ___________) that invalidate test results.
5. Accumulation of excess (A) ___________ fluid in the (B) ___________ cavity is called (C) ___________.
6. The patient must (A) ___________ ___________ material from (B) ___________ in the (C) ___________ (D) ___________ and not simply (E) ___________ into the container.
7. (A) ___________ urine specimen collection instructions must be accompanied by (B) ___________ instructions, preferably with (C) ___________.
8. A urine (A) ___________ ___________ test also requires collection of a (B) ___________ ___________ specimen, which is ideally collected at the (C) ___________ of urine collection (i.e., [D] ___________ ___________ into urine collection).
9. The (A) ___________ that causes TB is called an (B) ___________ ___________ ___________ (___________), and the (C) ___________ test for TB is often called an (D) ___________ culture.

KNOWLEDGE DRILL 13-2: SCRAMBLED WORDS

Unscramble the following words using the hints given in parentheses. Write the correct spelling of the scrambled word on the line next to it.

1. tonimica ___________ (fluid surrounding a fetus)
2. spiboy ___________ (take a tissue sample)
3. scoplebarneri ___________ (relating to the brain & spinal cord)
4. trueluc ___________ (grow microbes)
5. scirtag ___________ (relating to the stomach)
6. sademtirm ___________ (in the middle of urination)
7. lucoct ___________ (hidden)
8. ispartaes ___________ (they live off other organisms)

9. enoptralie ______________________ (relating to the abdominal cavity)
10. vistysintie ______________________ (microbe susceptibility)
11. visonlay ______________________ (of the joints)
12. dovedi ______________________ (urinated naturally)

KNOWLEDGE DRILL 13-3: CLEAN-CATCH URINE PROCEDURE RATIONALE

Match each of the following rationales to the steps of the *Clean-Catch Urine Collection Procedure for Women* (Procedure 13-2 in text) listed below. Place the appropriate letter in the Rationale column next to the step. (Rationales may be used more than once.)

Rationale

A. Aids in infection control.
B. Aids in infection control and helps avoid contamination of the site while cleaning.
C. Allows proper cleaning of the area.
D. Antiseptic solution in the wipe removes bacteria from area. Front-to-back motion carries bacteria away from the site.
E. Bringing the urine container into the stream without touching the genital area helps ensure sterility of the specimen. An adequate amount of urine is needed to perform the test.
F. Facilitates cleaning and downward flow of urine.
G. Follow facility protocol.
H. Only 30–100 mL urine is needed for the test.
I. Separation of the folds maintains site antisepsis. Voiding the first portion of urine into the toilet washes away the antiseptic and microbes remaining in the urinary opening.
J. The lid and container must remain sterile for accurate interpretation of results.
K. The lid and container must remain sterile, and specimen must be covered to maintain sterility and protect others from exposure to the contents.

Steps	Rationale
1. Wash hands thoroughly.	____
2. Remove the lid of the container, being careful not to touch the inside of the cover or the container.	____
3. Stand in a squatting position over the toilet.	____
4. Separate the folds of skin around the urinary opening.	____
5. Cleanse the area on either side and around the opening with the special wipes, using a fresh wipe for each area and wiping from front to back. Discard used wipes in the trash.	____
6. While keeping the skin folds separated, void into the toilet for a few seconds.	____
7. Touching only the outside and without letting it touch the genital area, bring the urine container into the urine stream until a sufficient amount of urine (30–100 mL) is collected.	____
8. Void the remaining urine into the toilet.	____

9. Cover the specimen with the lid provided, touching only the *outside* surfaces of the lid and container. ____
10. Clean any urine off the outside of the container with an antiseptic wipe. ____
11. Wash hands. ____
12. Hand specimen to phlebotomist or place where instructed if already labeled. ____

Skills Drills

SKILLS DRILL 13-1: REQUISITION ACTIVITY

The list of tests to choose from on a laboratory requisition includes the nonblood tests listed below. Write the meaning of the test abbreviation (or NA if not abbreviated) and the type of specimen required on the corresponding line.

Test	Abbreviation Meaning	Type of Specimen
1. AFB	____________	____________
2. *C. difficile*	____________	____________
3. CSF analysis	____________	____________
4. C-urea	____________	____________
5. Diphtheria culture	____________	____________
6. Guaiac	____________	____________
7. HCG	____________	____________
8. L/S ratio	____________	____________
9. Male fertility studies	____________	____________
10. O&P	____________	____________
11. Rapid strep	____________	____________
12. TB culture	____________	____________
13. UA C&S	____________	____________

SKILLS DRILL 13-2: WORD BUILDING

Divide each word below into all of its elements (parts); prefix (P), word root (WR), combining vowel (CV), and suffix (S). Write the word part, its definition, and the meaning of the word on the corresponding lines. If the word does not have a particular element, write NA (not applicable) in its place.

Example: gastric

Elements ______ / *gastr* / ___ / *ic*
P WR CV S

Definitions ______ / *stomach* / ___ / *pertaining*

Meaning: pertaining to the stomach

1. cerebrospinal

Elements ______ / ______ / ___ / ______
P WR CV S

Definitions ______ / ______ / ___ / ______

Meaning:

2. cytology

Elements ______ / ______ / ___ / ______
P WR CV S

Definitions ______ / ______ / ___ / ______

Meaning:

3. hemolytic

Elements ______ / ______ / ___ / ______ / ______
P WR CV WR S

Definitions ______ / ______ / ___ / ______ / ______

Meaning:

4. meningitis

Elements ______ / ______ / ___ / ______
P WR CV S

Definitions ______ / ______ / ___ / ______

Meaning:

5. nasopharynx

Elements ______ / ______ / ___ / ______
P WR CV S

Definitions ______ / ______ / ___ / ______

Meaning:

6. pericardial

Elements ______ / ______ / ___ / ______
P WR CV S

Definitions ______ / ______ / ___ / ______

Meaning:

SKILLS DRILL 13-3: 24-HOUR URINE COLLECTION PROCEDURE (Text Procedure 13-1)

Fill in the blanks with the missing information.

Steps	Explanation/Rationale
1. Void into toilet as usual upon awakening.	The bladder must be (A) ____________ when (B) ____________ starts. Urine voided is from the previous time period.
2. Note the (C) ____________ and date on the specimen label, place it on the container, and begin timing.	Timing (which should ideally start between 6 A.M. and 8 A.M.) is important. If urine is collected for a longer (D) ____________, period, results will be inaccurate. The label should be affixed to the container, not the lid.
3. Collect all urine voided for the next 24 hours.	Results are based on the (E) ____________ ____________ of urine produced in 24 hours.
4. (F) ____________ the specimen throughout the collection period if required.	Most specimens (except urate tests) require (G) ________________ to maintain analyte (H) ____________. The specimen container should be kept cool in a disposable ice chest, placed in the bathtub, for example.
5. When a bowel movement is anticipated, collect the urine specimen (I)________________________.	Prevents (J) ____________ contamination of the specimen.
6. Drink a normal amount of (K) ____________ unless instructed to do otherwise.	Prevents (L) ________________ and facilitates specimen collection.
7. Void one last time at the end of the 24 hours.	This specimen must be (M) ________________________ ____________.
8. Seal the container, place it in a portable cooler, and transport it to the laboratory (N) ____________.	Cooling and (O) ____________ delivery help protect the integrity of the specimen.

SKILLS DRILL 13-4: THROAT CULTURE COLLECTION PROCEDURE HIGHLIGHT SUMMARIES
(Text Procedure 13-4)

The following are summaries of *Throat Culture Specimen Collection Procedure* highlights. Fill in the blanks with the missing information.

1. The phlebotomist may wish to wear a (A) ____________ and goggles because throat culture collection will often cause the patient to have a gag reflex or (B) ____________.
2. Open container and remove swab in an (C) ____________ manner because (D) ____________ of the swab must be maintained for accurate (E) ________________ of results.
3. Stand back or to the (F) ____________ of the patient to help avoid (G) ____________ contact if the patient coughs.
4. Direct light onto the back of the throat using a small flashlight or other light source to illuminate areas of (H) ______________, ulceration, (I) ______________, or capsule formation.
5. Depress the tongue with a tongue depressor to help avoid touching other areas of the mouth and (J) ________________ the sample during collection.
6. Asking the patient to say "ah" raises the (K) ____________ (soft tissue hanging from the back of the throat) out of the way.
7. Swab both (L) ____________, the back of the throat, and any areas of ulceration, exudation, or inflammation, being careful not to touch the swab to the lips, (M) ____________, or uvula.
8. Touching the (N) ____________ can cause a (O) ____________ reflex.
9. Maintain tongue (P) ____________ position while removing the swab to prevent the tongue from contaminating the swab.
10. Place the swab back in the transport tube, embed in (Q) ____________, and secure cover to keep the microbes (R) ____________ until they can be cultured in the laboratory.

Crossword

ACROSS

1. Urine sample collection method
6. ____________ chloride
7. Grow microbes on nutrient media
8. Aspirated and examined to detect disease
9. Urine screening is performed to detect these
11. Specimens coughed up from deep in the lungs
12. Hormone in urine after conception (abbrev.)
15. Test on urine sample
17. Normal antigen found in amniotic fluid (abbrev.)
19. Most frequently analyzed nonblood fluid
20. ____________ syndrome
21. A sterile polyester-tipped collection device
22. Hidden blood in stool
23. ____________ and parasites
26. Related to the lung
27. Fluid secreted from glands in the mouth
29. Urinalysis (abbrev.)
31. Synovial fluid is found in this type of cavity
33. Urine specimen type that requires watching the clock
35. Amniotic test indicating fetal lung maturity (abbrev.)
36. Sperm-containing fluid
37. Fluid surrounding the fetus in the uterus

DOWN

1. Study of cells
2. Insert a tube through the urethra to collect urine
3. Person who performs chemistry tests
4. Pertaining to the stomach
5. Serum-like fluid
6. Feces
7. Fluid around the brain and spinal cord (abbrev., plural)
10. Throat culture to diagnose this bacterium
13. Test for hidden blood in feces
14. Type of urine specimen collected at any time
15. Common urinary tract ailment (abbrev.)
16. Viscous fluid found in joint cavities
18. Cells on the inside of the cheek
24. Type of steroid used to enhance people in sports
25. Liquid and semiliquid substances produced by the body
26. *Helicobacter* ____________
28. Urinate
30. Prescribed course of eating
32. Method of examination
34. Analysis using buccal cells from inside the cheek

Chapter Review Questions

1. In accepting a specimen for transport to the lab from a nursing unit, it is important to verify:
   a. billing code information.
   b. name of nurse requesting transport.
   c. patient identification information.
   d. physician requesting the test.

2. Which of the following can be detected by chemical analysis of a urine specimen?
   a. Clarity
   b. Crystals
   c. Glucose
   d. All of the above

3. Sputum specimens are used to detect:
   a. cystic fibrosis.
   b. pregnancy.
   c. recent drug use.
   d. tuberculosis.

4. This test is used to detect *Helicobacter pylori.*
   a. AFB
   b. C-UBT
   c. Guaiac
   d. NP culture

5. Synovial fluid is aspirated from the:
   a. heart.
   b. lungs.
   c. joints.
   d. stomach.

6. Pilocarpine is used in this test procedure.
   a. Bone marrow biopsy
   b. Gastric analysis
   c. CSF collection
   d. Sweat chloride

7. Urine cytology studies can be performed to detect:
   a. alpha-fetoprotein.
   b. cytomegalovirus.
   c. infertility.
   d. meningitis.

8. The specimen for this test requires stat handling and is typically collected by a physician in three sterile tubes.
   a. CSF analysis
   b. Gastric analysis
   c. Nasopharyngeal culture
   d. Suprapubic urine specimen

9. This test requires a 24-hour urine specimen.
   a. Creatinine clearance
   b. Glucose tolerance
   c. HCG detection
   d. Urine cytology

10. Which of the following would most likely lead to the repeat collection of a drug-screening specimen?
    a. pH is too low
    b. pH is too high
    c. SG is too low
    d. All of the above

11. A urine pregnancy test detects the presence of:
    a. AFP.
    b. DNA.
    c. HCG.
    d. UTI.

12. This type of sample can show evidence of long-term drug use.
    a. Breath
    b. Feces
    c. Hair
    d. Saliva

13. Which of the following urine specimens will normally have the highest specific gravity?
    a. First morning
    b. Midstream
    c. Random
    d. 24-hour

14. A urine sensitivity test:
    a. detects inflammatory disorders.
    b. exposes antibiotic susceptibility.
    c. identifies a microorganism.
    d. screens for illegal drug use.

15. Bone marrow samples are typically evaluated in:
    a. chemistry and microbiology.
    b. coagulation and blood bank.
    c. hematology and histology.
    d. serology and immunology.

CASE STUDIES

Case Study 13-1 CSF Specimen Handling

A nurse delivered three vials of CSF to the lab. A phlebotomist newly trained in specimen processing accepted the specimens from the nurse. The phlebotomist had never received CSF specimens before and was not sure what to do with them. She was extremely busy and her supervisor was at lunch, so she set the vials aside, intending to ask her supervisor what to do with them upon her return. The supervisor got called to an emergency meeting and did not return for several hours. The phlebotomist was so busy that she completely forgot about the CSF specimens until the physician called for the results on them. When he found out that the specimens had not been tested, he was furious. The specimens had to be recollected and the phlebotomist almost lost her job.

QUESTIONS

1. How could this incident have been prevented?
2. Why did the specimens have to be collected again?
3. How is a CSF specimen collected?

Case Study 13-2 Urine C&S Specimen Collection

Luann recently received on-the-job phlebotomy training. Today was the first day she was allowed to work alone. It was a busy day and patients were starting to stack up in the waiting area. One elderly woman needed a blood test and a urine C&S. Luann was good at drawing blood and liked doing it. She hated to instruct patients in urine collection, however. She drew the blood specimen, quickly bandaged the patient, and handed her a labeled urine collection container and several antiseptic wipes. She asked the patient if she had ever given a urine specimen before, and when the patient said yes, she showed her where the restroom was and told her that she should put the specimen on the counter when she was finished; then she could leave. She then called another patient in for a blood draw. The elderly woman came out of the restroom, set the specimen on the counter as she had been told, and left. Later that day, when things quieted down, Luann discovered that the patient had placed the antiseptic wipes in the urine container with the specimen. She was mad that the woman could be so foolish and also that she would have to call her, ask her to return to the lab, and instruct her in how to submit a new specimen.

QUESTIONS

1. Why would the patient make such a mistake if she had submitted a urine specimen before?
2. What should Luann have done that would have prevented the problem?

CHAPTER

14

Arterial Puncture Procedures

OBJECTIVES

Study the information in your textbook that corresponds to each objective to prepare yourself for the activities in this chapter.

1. Define the key terms and abbreviations listed at the beginning of this chapter.
2. State the primary reason for performing arterial punctures and identify the personnel who may be required to perform them.
3. Explain the purpose of collecting arterial blood gas (ABG) specimens and identify and describe commonly measured ABG parameters.
4. Identify the sites that can be used for arterial puncture, the criteria used for selection of the site, and the advantages and disadvantages of each site.
5. List equipment and supplies needed for arterial puncture.
6. Identify typical required and supplemental requisition information and describe patient assessment and preparation procedures, including the administration of local anesthetic, prior to drawing arterial blood gas specimens.
7. Explain the purpose of the modified Allen test, describe how it is performed, define what constitutes a positive or negative result, and give the procedure to follow for either result.
8. Describe the procedure for collecting radial arterial blood gas specimens and the role of the phlebotomist in other site collections.
9. List hazards and complications of arterial puncture, identify sampling errors that may affect the integrity of an arterial specimen, and describe the criteria for specimen rejection.

Matching

Use choices only once unless otherwise indicated.

MATCHING 14-1: KEY TERMS AND DESCRIPTIONS

Match each key term with the *best* description.

Key Terms

1. _____ Abducted
2. _____ ABGs
3. _____ Allen test
4. _____ Arteriospasm
5. _____ Brachial artery
6. _____ Collateral circulation
7. _____ Femoral artery
8. _____ FiO_2
9. _____ L/M
10. _____ Radial artery
11. _____ Steady state
12. _____ Ulnar artery

Descriptions

A. Area is supplied with blood from more than one artery
B. Artery located in the antecubital fossa near the insertion of the biceps muscle
C. Artery located in the groin, lateral to the pubic bone
D. Artery located on the little-finger side of the wrist
E. Artery located on the thumb side of the wrist
F. Fraction of inspired oxygen, as in oxygen therapy
G. Liters per minute, as in oxygen therapy
H. Out to the side, away from the body
I. Reflex or involuntary contraction of an artery
J. Stable condition with no exercise, suctioning, or respirator changes for 20 to 30 minutes
K. Test performed to assess collateral circulation before arterial puncture
L. Test used to assess a patient's oxygenation, ventilation, and acid–base balance

MATCHING 14-2: ARTERIES AND ADVANTAGES AND DISADVANTAGES

Match the arteries to the advantages and disadvantages associated with performing arterial punctures on them. Some advantages and disadvantages may have more than one choice.

Arteries

A. Radial
B. Brachial
C. Femoral

Advantages

1. _____ easy to compress after puncture
2. _____ fairly close to the surface of the skin
3. _____ has the best collateral circulation
4. _____ large and easy to palpate
5. _____ less chance of hematoma formation
6. _____ may be only choice during low cardiac output
7. _____ no major nerves or veins immediately adjacent
8. _____ preferred for collection of large volumes of blood

Disadvantages

1. _____ deeply located
2. _____ hardest to locate during low cardiac output
3. _____ increased chance of dislodging plaque
4. _____ increased risk of hematoma formation
5. _____ increased risk of infection
6. _____ lies close to a major vein
7. _____ lies close to the median nerve
8. _____ no underlying ligaments or bone
9. _____ poor collateral circulation
10. _____ small size requires more skill to puncture

Labeling Exercises

LABELING EXERCISE 14-1: ARM AND LEG ARTERIES (Text Figs. 14-2 and 14-3)

Identify each artery of the arm and leg identified by the numbered arrows and write the name on the corresponding numbered line below.

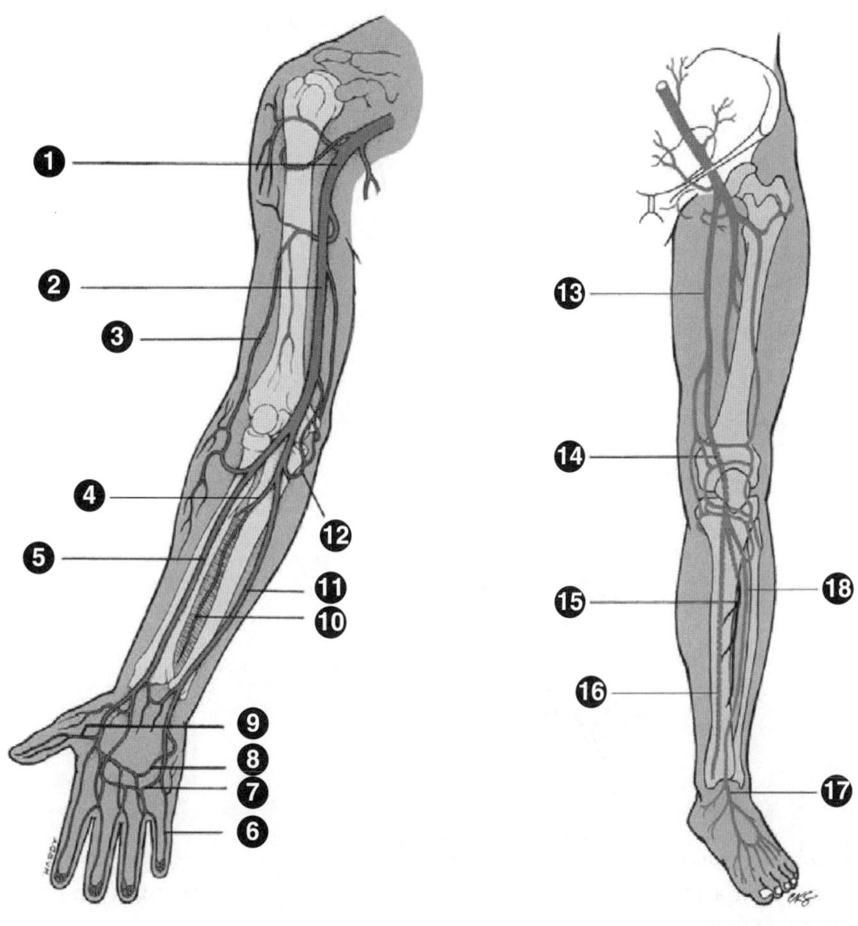

1. ______________________
2. ______________________
3. ______________________
4. ______________________
5. ______________________
6. ______________________
7. ______________________
8. ______________________
9. ______________________
10. ______________________
11. ______________________
12. ______________________
13. ______________________
14. ______________________
15. ______________________
16. ______________________
17. ______________________
18. ______________________

LABELING EXERCISE 14-2: ARTERIAL PUNCTURE SITES

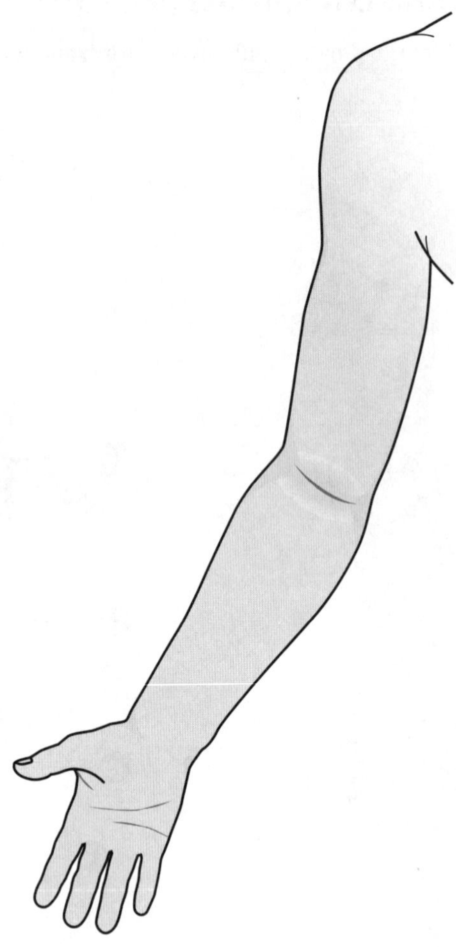

Draw X's on the approximate sites on the arm where arterial puncture is performed. Write #1 next to the X on the site that is the first choice for arterial puncture. Write the name of the first choice artery on line 1 below. Write the name of the other artery on line 2.

1. ______________________________

2. ______________________________

Knowledge Drills

KNOWLEDGE DRILL 14-1: CAUTION AND KEY POINT RECOGNITION

The following sentences are Caution or Key Point statements found throughout the Chapter 14 text. Using the TEXTBOOK, fill in the blanks with the missing information.

1. *Never* select a site in a limb with an (A) ____________ or (B) ____________. It is a patient's lifeline for (C) ____________ and should not be disturbed; also, venous and arterial blood (D) ____________ ____________ at the site.
2. *Never* use the (A) ____________ to (B) ____________, as it has a (C) ____________ that can be misleading.
3. *Do not* (A) ____________. (B) ____________ is painful and can cause (C) ____________ or (D) ____________ formation, or damage the artery.
4. *Never* allow the patient to (A) ____________ the (B) ____________. A patient may not (C) ____________ it firmly enough. In addition, *do not* replace use of (D) ____________ ____________ for the required length of time with the application of a pressure bandage.
5. *Never* leave the patient if the site is still (A) ____________. If (B) ____________ ____________ ____________ ____________ within a reasonable time, notify the patient's (C) ____________ or (D) ____________ of the problem.
6. According to CLSI, the (A) ____________ artery in children, especially infants, is not commonly used because it is (B) ____________ to (C) ____________ and lacks (D) ____________ ____________.

KNOWLEDGE DRILL 14-2: SCRAMBLED WORDS

Unscramble the following words, using the hints given in parentheses. Write the correct spelling of the scrambled word on the line next to it.

1. cudadebt ______________________________ (arm position for ABG collection)
2. narul ______________________________ (artery released first in an Allen test)
3. egxony ______________________________ (analyte measured by an ABG test)
4. eydats ______________________________ (patient state for accurate ABGs)
5. fiddemoi ______________________________ (changed from the original)
6. nivetonliat ______________________________ (air entering and leaving the lungs)
7. oltraclela ______________________________ (circulation requirement for arterial puncture)
8. slavogava ______________________________ (relating to a reaction by a particular nerve)
9. smearpotrisa ______________________________ (vessel reaction to arterial puncture)
10. tencheasti ______________________________ (a substance that dulls pain)
11. traleria ______________________________ (specimen required for ABGs)
12. vanigtee ______________________________ (Allen test result that means "choose another site")

KNOWLEDGE DRILL 14-3: HAZARDS AND COMPLICATIONS OF ARTERIAL PUNCTURE

List eight hazards or complications of arterial puncture.

1. ______
2. ______
3. ______
4. ______
5. ______
6. ______
7. ______
8. ______

KNOWLEDGE DRILL 14-4: SAMPLING ERRORS

List seven sampling errors associated with ABG collection.

1. ______
2. ______
3. ______
4. ______
5. ______
6. ______
7. ______

KNOWLEDGE DRILL 14-5: CRITERIA FOR SPECIMEN REJECTION

List eight criteria for specimen rejection and state how you would prevent such a rejection from happening.

Rejection Criteria	Prevention Tactic
1. ______________	______________
2. ______________	______________
3. ______________	______________
4. ______________	______________
5. ______________	______________
6. ______________	______________
7. ______________	______________
8. ______________	______________

KNOWLEDGE DRILL 14-6: COMMONLY MEASURED ABG ANALYTES (Text Table 14-1)

Fill in the blanks with the missing information.

Analyte	Normal Range	Description
PH	(A) ____________	A measure of the (B) ____________ or (C) ____________ of the blood; used to identify a condition such as acidosis or alkalosis.
(D) ____________	80–100 mm Hg	Partial pressure of (E) ____________ in arterial blood. A measure of how much (F) ____________ is dissolved in the blood. Indicates if (G) ____________ is adequate. Decreased (H) ____________ levels in the blood increase the respiration rate and vice versa.
$PaCO_2$	35–45 (I) ____________	Partial pressure of (J) ____________ ____________ in arterial blood. A measure of how much (K) ____________ ____________ is dissolved in the blood. Evaluates (L) ____________ function. Increased CO_2 levels in the blood increase the (M) ____________ rate and vice versa. *Respiratory* disturbances alter $PaCO_2$ levels.
(N) ____________	22–26 mEq/L	(O) ____________. A measure of the amount of (P) ____________ in the blood. Evaluates the bicarbonate buffer system of the kidneys. *Metabolic* and *respiratory* disturbances alter HCO_3 levels.
O_2 saturation	97%–100%	Oxygen saturation. The percent of (Q) ____________ bound to (R) ____________. Determines if (S) ____________ is carrying the amount of (T) ____________ it is capable of carrying.
Base excess (or deficit)	(−2)–(+2) mEq/L	A calculation of the (U) ____________ part of acid–base balance based on the PCO_2, HCO_3, and hemoglobin.

Skills Drills

SKILLS DRILL 14-1: REQUISITION ACTIVITY

A physician sends a patient to a hospital outpatient lab with the stat order shown below.

Lic.# 000000

John Chursdt, MD
2011 Happy Street
Suite 9
Any Town USA

Name *Jane Doe* Age *66*

Address ______ Date *Sept. 19, 2011*

℞

ABGs & LYtes

Patient has hx COPD
WBC drawn yesterday elevated

Signature *JChursdt, MD*

1. What effect does a high WBC have on ABGs? ______

2. How many draws will it take to collect specimens for all of the ordered tests? ______

3. What type of syringe should be used to collect the ABG specimen? ______

4. How should the specimen(s) be transported? ______

SKILLS DRILL 14-2: WORD BUILDING

Divide each word into all of its elements (parts); prefix (P), word root (WR), combining vowel (CV), and suffix (S). Write the word part, its definition, and the meaning of the word on the corresponding lines. If the word does not have a particular element, write NA (not applicable) in its place.

Example: asepsis

Elements *a* / *sep* / ______ / *sis*
P WR CV S

Definitions *without* / *pathogenic organisms* / ______ / *condition of*

Meaning: condition of being without pathogen organism

1. acidosis

   Elements ______ / ______ / ______ / ______
   P WR CV S

   Definitions ______ / ______ / ______ / ______

   General Meaning:

2. anaerobic

   Elements ______ / ______ / ______ / ______
   P WR CV S

   Definitions ______ / ______ / ______ / ______

   General Meaning:

3. anesthetic

   Elements ______ / ______ / ______ / ______
   P WR CV S

   Definitions ______ / ______ / ______ / ______

   General Meaning:

4. arteriospasm

   Elements ______ / ______ / ______ / ______
   P WR CV S

   Definitions ______ / ______ / ______ / ______

   General Meaning:

5. brachial

   Elements ______ / ______ / ______ / ______
   P WR CV S

   Definitions ______ / ______ / ______ / ______

   General Meaning:

6. femoral

   Elements ______ / ______ / ______ / ______
   P WR CV S

   Definitions ______ / ______ / ______ / ______

   General Meaning:

7. hypodermic

   Elements ______ / ______ / ______ / ______
   P WR CV S

   Definitions ______ / ______ / ______ / ______

   General Meaning:

8. radial

Elements	______ /	______ /	______ /	______
	P	WR	CV	S
Definitions	______ /	______ /	______ /	______

General Meaning:

SKILLS DRILL 14-3: MODIFIED ALLEN TEST PROCEDURE (Text Procedure 14-1)

Fill in the blanks with the missing information.

Step	Explanation/Rationale
1. Have the patient make a tight fist.	A tight fist partially blocks (A) ______ ______, causing temporary (B) ______ until the hand is opened.
2. Use the middle and index fingers of both hands to apply pressure to the patient's wrist, compressing both the (C) ______ and (D) ______ arteries at the same time.	Pressure over both arteries is needed to (E) ______ blood flow, which is required to be able to assess (F) ______ ______ when pressure is released.
3. While maintaining pressure, have the patient open the hand slowly. It should appear (G) ______ or drained of color.	(H) ______ appearance of the hand verifies temporary blockage of both arteries. Note: The patient must not (I) ______ the fingers when opening the hand, as this can cause (J)______ blood flow and (K) ______ of results.
4. Lower the patient's hand and release pressure on the (L) ______ artery only.	The (M) ______ artery is released while the (N) ______ is still obstructed to determine if it will be able to provide blood flow should the (O) ______ artery be injured during ABG collection.
5. Assess results: *Positive Allen test result:* The hand (P) ______ ______ or returns to normal color within 15 seconds. *Negative Allen test result:* The hand (S) ______ ______ ______ ______ or return to normal color within 15 seconds.	A positive test result indicates return of blood to the hand via the (Q) ______ artery and the (R) ______ of collateral circulation. If the Allen test is positive, proceed with ABG collection. A negative test result indicates inability of the (T) ______ artery to adequately supply blood to the hand and therefore the (U) ______ of collateral circulation. If the Allen test result is negative, the (V) ______ artery should not be used and another site must be selected.
6. Record the results on the (W) ______.	Verification that the Allen test was performed.

SKILLS DRILL 14-4: RADIAL ABG PROCEDURE (Text Procedure 14-3)

Fill in the blanks with the missing information.

Step	Explanation/Rationale
1. (A) ______________ and accession test request.	The requisition must be reviewed for completeness of information (see Chapter 8, "Venipuncture Procedure," step 1) and required collection (B) ______________, such as oxygen delivery system, and (C) ______________ or L/M.
2. Approach, identify and prepare patient.	Correct approach to the patient, identification, and preparation are essential (see Chapter 8, "Venipuncture Procedure," step 2). Preparing the patient by explaining the procedure in a calm and reassuring manner encourages cooperation and reduces apprehension. ((D) ______________ due to anxiety, breath-holding, or crying can alter test results.)
3. Check for sensitivities to latex and other substances.	Increasing numbers of individuals are allergic to latex, (E) ______________, and other substances.
4. Assess (G) ______________ ______________, verify collection requirements, and record required information.	Required collection conditions must be met and must not have changed for (H) ______________ prior to collection. Test results can be meaningless or misinterpreted and patient care compromised if they have not been met. The patient's temperature, respiratory rate, and FiO_2 affect blood gas (I) ______________ and must be recorded along with other required information.
5. (J) ______________ hands and put on gloves.	Proper hand hygiene plays a major role in (K) ______________ ______________, protecting the phlebotomist, patient, and others from contamination. Gloves provide a barrier to blood-borne pathogen exposure. Gloves may be put on at this point or later, depending on hospital protocol.
6. Assess (L) ______________ circulation.	(M) ______________ circulation must be verified by either the modified (N) ______________ test, ultrasonic flow indicator, or both. Proceed if result is (O) ______________; choose another site if (P) ______________.

7. Position arm, ask patient to (Q) __________ wrist.	The arm should be (R) __________ with the palm up and the wrist (S) __________ approximately 30 degrees to stretch and fix the soft tissues over the firm ligaments and bone. (Avoid (T) __________, as it can eliminate a palpable pulse.)
8. Locate the radial artery and clean the site.	The (U) __________ __________ is used to locate the radial pulse (V) __________ to the skin crease on the (W) __________ side of the wrist; palpate it to determine size, depth, and direction. An arterial site is typically cleaned with alcohol or another suitable antiseptic and must not be touched again until the phlebotomist is ready to access the artery.
9. Administer local (X) __________ (optional).	(See Procedure 14-2.) Document anesthetic application on the requisition.
10. Prepare equipment and clean gloved nondominant finger.	Assemble ABG equipment and set the (Y) __________ __________ to the proper fill level if applicable. Gloves must be put on at this point if this has not already been done, and the nondominant finger cleaned so that it does not contaminate the site when relocating the pulse before needle entry.
11. Pick up equipment and uncap and inspect needle.	The syringe is held in the dominant hand as if holding a (Z) __________. The needle must be inspected for defects, and replaced if any are found.
12. Relocate radial artery and warn patient of (AA) __________ __________.	The artery is relocated by placing the nondominant index finger directly over the (BB) __________. The patient is warned to prevent a (CC) __________ __________ and asked to relax the wrist to help ensure a smooth needle entry.
13. Insert the needle at a 30- to 45-degree angle, slowly direct it toward the (DD) __________, and stop when a (EE) __________ of blood appears.	A needle inserted at a 30- to 45-degree angle 5 to 10 mm (FF) __________ to the finger that is over the pulse should contact the artery directly under that finger. When the artery is entered, a (GG) __________ of blood normally appears in the needle hub or syringe. Note: If a needle smaller than 23-gauge is used, it may be necessary to pull gently on the syringe plunger to obtain blood flow.

14. Allow the syringe to fill to the proper level.	Blood will normally fill the syringe under its own (HH) ____________, which is an indication that the specimen is indeed arterial blood. (See exception in step 13.)
15. Place gauze, remove needle, activate safety feature, and (II) ____________ ____________.	A clean, folded gauze square is placed over the site so firm manual pressure can be applied by the (JJ) ____________ immediately upon needle removal and for 3 to 5 minutes thereafter. The needle safety device must be activated as soon as possible in order to prevent an accidental needlestick.
16. Remove and discard syringe needle.	For safety reasons, the specimen must not be transported with the needle attached to the syringe. The needle must be removed and discarded in the sharps container with one hand while site pressure is applied with the other.
17. Expel (KK) ____________ ____________, cap syringe, mix and label specimen.	(LL) ____________ ____________ in the specimen can affect test results and must be expelled per manufacturer's instructions. The specimen must be capped to maintain (MM) ____________ conditions, mixed thoroughly by inversion or rotating to prevent clotting, labeled with required information, and, if applicable, placed in coolant to protect analytes from the effects of cellular metabolism.
18. Check patient's arm and apply bandage.	The site is checked for swelling or bruising after pressure has been applied for 3 to 5 minutes. If the site is warm and appears normal, pressure is applied for 2 more minutes, after which the (NN) ____________ is checked (OO) ____________ to the site to confirm normal blood flow. If pulse and site are normal, a pressure bandage is applied and the time at which it should be removed is noted. Note: If the pulse is weak or absent, the patient's nurse or physician must be notified immediately.
19. Dispose of used and contaminated materials, remove gloves, and sanitize hands.	Used and contaminated items must be disposed of per facility protocol. Gloves must be removed and hands sanitized as an (PP) ____________ ____________ ____________.
20. Thank patient, and transport specimen to the lab (QQ) ____________.	Thanking the patient is courteous and professional behavior. Prompt delivery of the specimen to the lab protects specimen (RR) ____________.

Crossword Exercise

ACROSS

1. Involuntary arterial contraction
5. With air
7. Mass of blood; often clotted
9. Concerning palm of the hand
10. Type of microbe
11. ABG collection equipment
12. The preferred one for ABG is 22-gauge
13. Hit the artery, see a ____________
14. Preferred point of entry
17. Allen test checks for ____________ flow
18. Syringe part capped after collection
21. Arterial blood gas (abbrev.)
23. Test for collateral flow
25. Contaminant of ABGs
26. ABG component measured
27. Allen test result

DOWN

1. Without air
2. Another name for clot
3. Protective equipment (abbrev.)
4. First-choice ABG site
6. Second-choice AB site
7. Anticoagulant for ABGs
8. Abrupt loss of consciousness response
15. Lidocaine, for one
16. Artery in the wrist
19. Hold the ABG syringe like a ____________
20. Unacceptable way to find vein
22. PPEs for hands
23. 30- to 45-degree ____________ for ABGs
24. Anesthetic used to ____________ site

Chapter Review Questions

1. Which of the following personnel may be required to perform arterial puncture?
   a. EMTs
   b. MTs
   c. Phlebotomists
   d. All of the above

2. O_2 saturation measures the:
   a. alkalinity of the blood plasma.
   b. amount of oxygen dissolved in the plasma.
   c. oxygen pressure in the lungs.
   d. percent of oxygen bound to hemoglobin.

3. Which is the first-choice artery for ABG collection?
   a. Brachial
   b. Femoral
   c. Radial
   d. Ulnar

4. Which of the following is the most important criterion for selecting an artery for ABG collection provided that there is no other reason to avoid the site?
   a. Collateral circulation
   b. Depth of the artery
   c. Dominance of the arm
   d. Strength of the pulse

5. The anticoagulant used in ABG specimen collection is:
   a. EDTA.
   b. heparin.
   c. potassium oxalate.
   d. sodium citrate.

6. In addition to identification information, which of the following is typically documented before ABG specimen collection?
   a. FiO_2 or L/M
   b. History of smoking
   c. Room temperature
   d. All of the above

7. A phlebotomist must collect an ABG specimen when the patient is breathing room air. The patient has just been taken off the ventilator when the phlebotomist arrives. When can the phlebotomist draw the ABG specimen?
   a. After 1 hour
   b. Immediately
   c. In 5 to 10 minutes
   d. In 20 to 30 minutes

8. A phlebotomist has a request to collect an ABG specimen on a patient. The patient has a positive Allen test on the right arm. What should the phlebotomist do?
   a. Collect the specimen by capillary puncture.
   b. Collect the specimen from the right radial artery.
   c. Collect the specimen from the right ulnar artery.
   d. Perform the Allen test on the left arm.

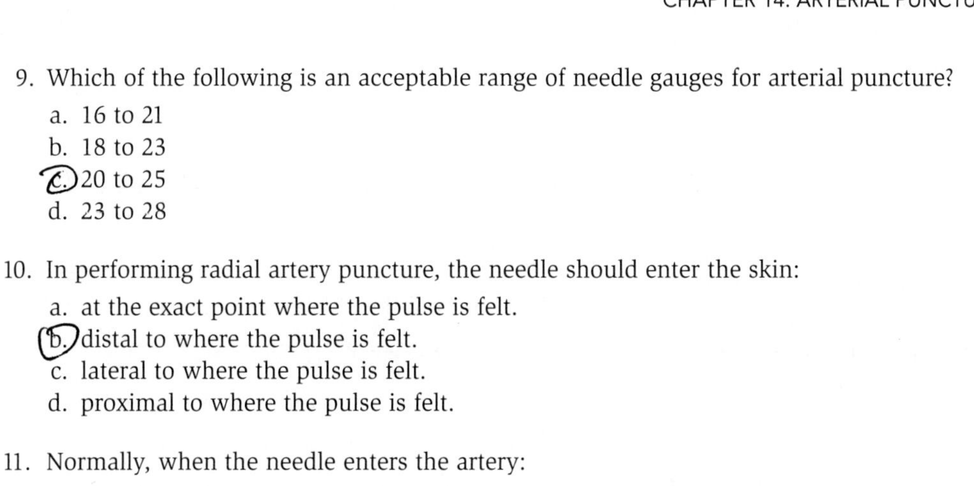

9. Which of the following is an acceptable range of needle gauges for arterial puncture?
   a. 16 to 21
   b. 18 to 23
   c. 20 to 25
   d. 23 to 28

10. In performing radial artery puncture, the needle should enter the skin:
    a. at the exact point where the pulse is felt.
    b. distal to where the pulse is felt.
    c. lateral to where the pulse is felt.
    d. proximal to where the pulse is felt.

11. Normally, when the needle enters the artery:
    a. a flash of blood appears in the syringe.
    b. the syringe plunger starts to vibrate.
    c. you may hear a soft swishing sound.
    d. all of the above can happen.

12. An ABG specimen is most likely to be rejected if it:
    a. arrives at the lab 20 minutes after collection.
    b. contains only around 2 milliliters of blood.
    c. is collected in a glass syringe.
    d. is determined to be QNS.

13. Which of the following is the best way to tell that the specimen you are collecting is in fact arterial blood?
    a. A flash of blood appeared in the syringe on needle entry.
    b. Blood pulsed into the syringe under its own power.
    c. The color of the blood is bright cherry-red.
    d. There is no way to tell for certain.

14. A single routine arterial specimen for both ABG and electrolyte testing should be transported:
    a. at room temperature.
    b. green-top tube.
    c. on ice.
    d. STAT.

15. The risk of hematoma associated with arterial puncture is greatest if:
    a. a large-diameter needle is used.
    b. the patient is elderly.
    c. the patient is on a blood thinner.
    d. all of the above.

CASE STUDIES

Case Study 14-1 Modified Allen Test and ABG Specimen Collection

A phlebotomist has a request to collect a STAT ABG specimen on a patient. He had collected an ABG specimen the night before from the same patient on the same arm, and since the patient had a positive modified Allen test then, he skips the Allen test now to save time. As he is preparing to insert the needle, the patient's nurse enters the room and tells him to stop. She tells him that the patient does not have adequate collateral circulation in that arm and he must not collect the specimen there.

QUESTIONS

1. What error did the phlebotomist make?
2. How could the error have been avoided?
3. What could have caused the change in collateral circulation?

Case Study 14-2 ABG Hazards and Complications

A phlebotomist had an order to collect STAT ABG and electrolyte specimens from a patient in the ICU. The patient was having difficulty breathing when the phlebotomist arrived. There was an IV in the patient's right arm, so the phlebotomist performed the Allen test on the left arm. The test result was positive, so the phlebotomist proceeded to collect the specimen from the radial artery of that arm. He had to redirect the needle several times before dark bluish-red blood finally pulsed into the syringe. When the syringe was filled to the proper level, he withdrew the needle and held pressure over the site. As he was attempting to cap the syringe, the cap dropped into the patient's bed covers, so the phlebotomist asked the patient to hold pressure while he retrieved it. Later, when he went to check the arm, a large hematoma had formed at the collection site. When he checked the patient's pulse below the collection site, it was so weak he could barely feel it.

QUESTIONS

1. What could have caused the weak pulse and what should the phlebotomist do about it?
2. What error did the phlebotomist make that contributed to hematoma formation?
3. What would cause the specimen to be bluish red?
4. How can the phlebotomist be certain that the specimen is arterial blood?

UNIT IV CROSSWORD EXERCISE

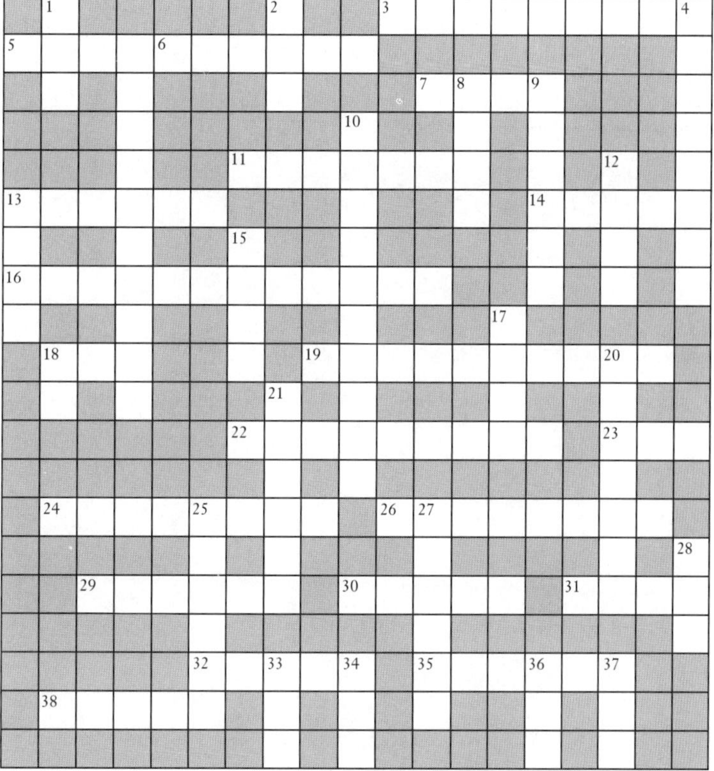

ACROSS

3. Term applied to urine collected in the middle of urination
5. Determines compatibility of blood for transfusion
7. Activated partial thromboplastin time (abbrev.)
11. With air
13. *Hyponatremia* means that this substance in the blood is decreased
14. Test for collateral flow
16. Involuntary contraction of an artery
18. Ailment caused by microorganisms somewhere in the urinary system
19. Machine used to spin blood tubes at high rpm
22. An O&P test can detect these
23. Evacuated tube with separator gel (abbrev.)
24. Type of fluid that surrounds a fetus in the uterus
26. A secret code that allows access to a computer system
29. Type of swab collected from the inside of the cheek
30. Key pushed in sending data to the processor
31. Image on a computer screen that represents a program or function
32. Type of testing done on the Cholestech instrument
35. Networking device customized to the tasks of routing and forwarding information
38. Iontophoresis is used to stimulate production of this substance

DOWN

1. Agent found in blood culture (BC) bottles to inhibit microorganism growth (abbrev.)
2. Test used to diagnose problems of carbohydrate metabolism
4. Intended to assist memory
6. Microorganisms or their toxins in the blood
8. Often called alternate-site testing
9. Another name for central processing
10. Type of circulation in which more than one artery supplies blood to an area
12. Sets standards for laboratory medicine (abbrev.)
13. Immediately
15. ____________ agglutinins
17. Point at which the needle will actually enter the skin
18. Analysis of urine (abbrev.)
20. Type of fluid collected from the stomach
21. Artery located at the thumb side of the wrist
25. Hidden
27. Brachial or radial
28. A buccal swab is used for this analysis
33. Tube used for separating plasma and free-flowing cells
34. These are special NIDA requirements for this urine test
36. Amount of time it takes from collection to results
37. Main processor memory (abbrev.)